Homosexuality and the Mental Health Professions

Committee on Human Sexuality
Group for the Advancement of Psychiatry

Bertram H. Schaffner, M.D., *Chair*

Paul L. Adams, M.D.

Jennifer I. Downey, M.D.

Jack Drescher, M.D. *(Chair-elect)*

Richard C. Friedman, M.D.

Joan A. Lang, M.D.

Joseph P. Merlino, M.D.

Harris Peck, M.D. *(deceased)*

Richard A. Friedman, M.D., *Consultant*

Pauline Quirion, *Consultant*

Christina Sekaer, M.D., *Consultant*

Martha Bird, M.D., *Fellow*

John Burton, M.D., *Fellow*

Justin Richardson, M.D., *Fellow*

Gwer Zornberg, M.D., *Fellow*

Cynthia Vitko, M.D., *Ginsburg Fellow Representative*

Homosexuality and the Mental Health Professions
The Impact of Bias

*formulated by
the Committee on Human Sexuality*

❧

GROUP FOR THE ADVANCEMENT OF PSYCHIATRY
REPORT NO. 144

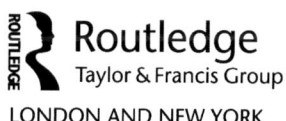
Routledge
Taylor & Francis Group
LONDON AND NEW YORK

First published 2000 by The Analytic Press, Inc.

Published 2014 by Routledge

2 Park Square, Milton Park, Abingdon, Oxfordshire OX14 4RN

711 Third Avenue, New York, NY 10017

First issued in paperback 2014

Routledge is an imprint of the Taylor & Francis Group, an informa business

© 2000 Group for the Advancement of Psychiatry
All rights reserved. No part of this book may be reproduced in any form: by photostat, microform, retrieval system, or any other means, without the prior written permission of the publisher.

Typeset in Trump Mediaeval by CompuDesign

Library of Congress Cataloging-in-Publication Data

Homosexuality and the mental health professions : the impact of bias / formulated by the Group for the Advancement of Psychiatry
    p.   cm.
Includes bibliographic references and index.
ISBN 978-0-88163-318-4 (hbk)
ISBN 978-1-13800-556-3 (pbk)
   1. Homosexuality. 2. Gays-Mental health services. 3. Prejudices.
4. Homophobia. I. Group for the Advancement of Psychiatry
[DNLM: 1. Homosexuality. 2. Attitude of Health Personnel.
3. Interpersonal Relations. 4. Mental Health Services. 5. Prejudice
HQ 76 H7675 2000]
RC558.H653 2000
362.2'64-dc21
99-059816

Contents

	Preface	*vii*
	Acknowledgments	*xvii*
1	Dimensions of Antihomosexual Bias	1
2	AHB in the Clinical Setting	25
3	The Impact of AHB on Supervision and Professional Training	55
4	Legal Aspects of Antihomosexual Bias and Mental Health	77
5	HIV and AHB in Mental Health	91
	References	*107*
	Index	*125*

Preface

The Group for the Advancement of Psychiatry And Its Past Reports Relating To Homosexuality

Historical GAP Positions on Social Issues Related to This Monograph

The Group for the Advancement of Psychiatry (GAP) was founded shortly after World War II in 1946 by young psychiatrists just returned from the war and impatient with the traditionalism of the American Psychiatric Association at that time. GAP's intended purpose was to produce position statements on relevant and controversial psychiatric issues. GAP reports were concise, published soon after they were written, and widely respected and influential. Possibly because of the profound social changes that followed World War II, both the profession and the public were ready to accept revisions of traditional psychiatric attitudes and practices. This monograph, *Homosexuality and the Mental Health Professions: The Impact of*

Bias, is in the tradition of a number of GAP publications dealing with bias, discrimination, and human sexuality.

GAP's formulated policy to discuss controversial psychosocial issues was announced in 1950, in the Committee on Social Issues' Report, *The Social Responsibility of Psychiatry, A Statement of Orientation* (The Group for the Advancement of Psychiatry, 1950b). In that report, the Committee noted that two factors had been influential in causing neglect of social problems by psychiatry: the role of prejudice in determining attitudes toward social problems and the sparse knowledge about the relationship between society and personality. In that pioneering document, the Committee on Social Issues emphasized the social responsibility of psychiatry. It made a number of suggestions for broadening the conceptual framework of psychiatry to include

> redefinition of the concept of mental illness, emphasizing those dynamic principles which pertain to the person's interaction with society . . . examination of the social factors which contribute to the causation of mental illness and also influence its course and outcome . . . consideration of the specific group psychological phenomena which are relevant, in a positive sense, to community mental health . . . the development of criteria for social action, relevant to the promotion of individual and community mental health [p. 5].

The Psychiatric Aspects of School Desegregation (The Group for the Advancement of Psychiatry, 1957), also produced by the Committee on Social Issues, addressed the issue of racial prejudice, around which there has been intense and ongoing conflict in American history. The following paragraph from the School Desegregation Report illustrates the way that GAP attempted to integrate psychosocial perceptions in the areas of both racial and sexual prejudice into individual and group psychodynamic theories:

On the deepest personal level, prejudices and their supporting myths can be understood as a means of maintaining feelings of self-esteem and security. In this sense they serve a defensive function. Many people of any race have acute doubts about their own worth, their adequacy in their sexual roles, and their acceptability as members of their groups. Turning attention to others' deficiencies permits one to remove the focus from fear and misgivings about oneself. Relief from intolerable feelings of self-contempt may be sought unconsciously by turning the hatred away from the despised part of oneself onto another person or group who, by the distortion of racial mythology, can represent the bad self. A down-graded minority, then, can become the source of a somewhat illusory security about oneself . . . the basis that "I am better than they are. . . ." But guilt feelings with associated anxiety are a frequent price for whatever psychological gains may come from such defensive dealing with inner conflicts. The use of the myth as a defense against insecurity, therefore, is self-defeating for it not only fails to reach a realistic solution of the original difficulty but also increases the original burden of guilt. The well-known vicious circle of anxiety, defense, increased anxiety, and increased defensiveness may then ensue [p. 167].

These two GAP monographs provide much of the framework within which this report is to be understood. Also important, however, have been GAP's previous discussions of human sexuality. In 1950, GAP published its first such report, *Psychiatrically Deviated Sex Offenders*, (The Group for the Advancement of Psychiatry, 1950a), written by the Committee on Forensic Psychiatry. The Committee's intent was to bring an end to the use of traditional stereotyping and unclear legal terms and to bring a fuller measure of psychiatric understanding of sexual behavior to the court system. It stated:

The Committee cautions against the use of this appellation "psychopath" in the law on several grounds. There is still little agreement on the part of psychiatrists as to the precise meaning of the term. Furthermore, the term has no dynamic significance. The Committee believes that in statutes the use of technical psychiatric terms should be avoided whenever possible. Psychiatric knowledge and terminology are in a state of flux. Once having become a part of public law such a term obtains a fixity unresponsive to newer scientific knowledge and applications [p. 1].

Despite the Committee's recommendation, in the *DSM-I* (American Psychiatric Association, 1952), which was shortly to follow, homosexuality was conceptualized as a form of psychopathic deviance.

GAP continued to focus on clinical psychiatric issues in human sexuality in later reports, for example: 1) *Assessment of Sexual Function: A Guide to Interviewing* (The Group for the Advancement of Psychiatry, 1973), formulated by the Committee on Medical Education, 2) *Psychiatry and Sex Psychopath Legislation: The 30's to the 80's* (The Group for the Advancement of Psychiatry, 1977), formulated by the Committee on Psychiatry and the Law; and 3) *Crises of Adolescence: Teenage Pregnancy: Impact on Adolescent Development*, formulated by the Committee on Adolescence (The Group for the Advancement of Psychiatry, 1986).

The earliest GAP publication to focus explicitly on sexual orientation was *Homosexuality with Particular Emphasis on This Problem in Governmental Agencies* (The Group for the Advancement of Psychiatry, 1955), formulated by the Committee on Cooperation with Governmental [Federal] Agencies. The Committee hoped that their scientific discussion of what they considered a frequently misunderstood condition might "result in a more effective appraisal and management of the practical problems that homosexuality creates in society in general and in Governmental agencies ... in particular" (p. 1).

The stated purpose of that report was "to define and describe homosexual behavior and homosexuality from a medical and social point of view in accordance with scientific principles" (p. 1). Consistent with prevailing psychiatric opinion of that time, the Committee responsible for the report identified homosexuality as a treatable illness, meaning that a person's homosexual orientation could be changed to a heterosexual one, and that it is

> a form of sexual perversion . . . psychological in origin [with] no valid evidence that homosexuality is inherited. Homosexuality is an arrest at, or a regression to, an immature level of psychosexual development. While the treatment of homosexuality is difficult and time-consuming, success has been reported. Psychotherapy offers the best chance of success, particularly in the turbulent transition period from adolescence to maturity wherein sexual goals have not been finally established [p. 6].

The report questioned the prevailing view that people's homosexual orientation posed high security risks due to their "lack of emotional stability . . . and the weakness of their moral fiber" and cautioned against the pursuit of "witch hunts" (p. 6). In closing, the Committee observed, "In the governmental setting as well as in civilian life, homosexuals have functioned with distinction, and without disruption of morale and efficiency. Problems of social maladaptive behavior, such as homosexuality, therefore need to be examined on an individual basis, considering the place and circumstances, rather than from inflexible rules" (p. 6).

In the middle of this century, scientists, scholars, and researchers in biology, biochemistry, endocrinology, ethology, evolutionary studies, experimental psychology, genetics, history, literary theory, neuroanatomy, religion, the social sciences, and philosophy began the process of advancing alternative models of homosexuality (Kinsey, Pomeroy, and

Martin, 1948; Friedman, 1988; McWhirter, Sanders, and Reinisch, 1990; Cabaj and Stein, 1996; Drescher, 1998b) opened up new knowledge about homosexuality and raised new questions that were not considered by psychiatrists in 1955. However, taken in its historical context, the 1955 GAP Monograph strongly argued against commonly accepted negative stereotypes that depicted a homosexual orientation prejudicially. It is uncertain what influence this report had on the implementation of antihomosexual policies of US governmental agencies. Of note, brief mention was also made of the topic of homosexuality in the *Sex and the College Student* (The Group for the Advancement of Psychiatry, 1960).

In contrast to directly addressing the issue of homosexuality, *The Educated Woman: Prospects and Problems* (The Group for the Advancement of Psychiatry, 1975), formulated by the Committee on the College Student, mentioned the topic as a footnote: "In the ensuing discussion we have primarily focused on heterosexual relationships because, besides being statistically most likely, they inevitably highlight issues relating to gender differences" (p. 188). They went on to state:

> Most individuals will opt for a heterosexual orientation, but for some a homosexual orientation may represent the orientation of choice. In either case the opportunity exists to learn how one's self concept, gender identity, and sexual responsiveness work in actual practice. In arriving at an adult sexual orientation, patterns of sexual relationships, both heterosexual and homosexual, may become exceedingly complex and will inevitably be affected by earlier developmental events, identification, and conflicts. . . . No single life style can be presumed a priori to be "healthier" or "more adaptive" for all persons. What is adaptive may not only differ from one person to another, but may also change for any given person as development proceeds throughout the life cycle [p. 189].

In 1990, fifteen years later, *Psychotherapy with College Students* (The Group for the Advancement of Psychiatry, 1990), formulated by the same Committee on the College Student, did discuss gay and lesbian students in the section, "Some Special Student Populations." In that report, the Committee more openly specified student problems to include 1) recognition and acceptance of sexual identity and orientation, 2) difficulties in establishing stable love relationships, and 3) managing relations with fellow students. Special attention was given to concerns of gay and lesbian students seeking psychotherapy in the college mental health services:

> Some gay students feel that they would prefer to work with a therapist who is openly gay, because no matter what the therapist claims, such students are suspicious that a therapist, presumably heterosexual, will be critical of their homosexuality. Most, however, are willing to work with any therapist who is nonjudgmental and accepting of the student's homosexual orientation. In confirming this acceptance, therefore, it is important for the therapist to be careful about asking questions that can be "heard" by the student as suggesting or urging heterosexual behavior. As gay students become more open about their orientation, they may become less conflicted about seeking therapy for whatever reasons, but they may also be more influenced by political positions of the campus gay organization [p. 119].

Fear of AIDS, problems with family, and discomfort with their own homosexuality were identified as common concerns in these students. The report was generally supportive of lesbian and gay students' efforts to find a healthy expression of their sexual orientation. Although it had been previously recognized that psychiatrists should come to terms with their own biases before they can successfully treat members of the other sex or of different races or other minority groups, that monograph was the first to call attention to the issue of antihomosexual bias (AHB), often referred to as "homophobia" in therapy.

The tragic emergence in 1981 of the AIDS epidemic made it obvious that antihomosexual bias not only impeded adequate care of AIDS patients, but also prevented educational measures and interfered with rapid governmental funding for medical research. The compelling practical need to better understand the nature of AHB and to reduce its impact both in the larger social picture and in the specific area of clinical psychiatry is the principal topic of this monograph.

Since Weinberg's (1972) definition of the term homophobia, the scientific and theoretical literature on the subject of AHB has grown (Boswell, 1980; Marmor, 1980; De Cecco, 1985; Herek and Glunt, 1988; Herek, 1990; Herek and Berrill, 1992; Abelove, Barale, and Halperin, 1993; Domenici and Lesser, 1995; Cabaj and Stein, 1996). Studies have concentrated on AHB's presence in specific groups and professions, such as government, business, law, and various branches of medicine. This report, however, is among the first to address the question of AHB specifically within psychiatric practice, training, and professional relationships. This report also raises questions about the adequacy of current knowledge and training of psychotherapists in the areas of sexual orientation and the impact of AHB in the treatment setting.

Background of the GAP Committee on Human Sexuality

The GAP Committee on Human Sexuality was created in 1989. Founding members of the Committee were influenced by the work of Rieker and Carmen (1984), who taught how to effectively combat prejudice through fostering attitude reassessment and modification. Their approach emphasized that overcoming prejudice was best done in small group settings in which conflicts about sex roles, gender identity, moral values, and other areas could be openly discussed.

Two GAP members, Dr. John Spiegel and Dr. Bertram Schaffner, were eager to find a way to extend these principles to the area of bias about homosexuality. They felt that AHB was as pervasive in the medical profession as it was in the general population and that it was usually ignored in medical and psychiatric education. They requested that the officers of GAP consider forming a new committee whose initial task would be to take up this issue. GAP's positive response was consistent with its commitment to open discussion of subjects that have been traditionally avoided in the psychiatric community.

At a GAP plenary session, speakers discussed problems faced by lesbian and gay psychiatrists. They reported that considerable numbers of gay and lesbian psychiatrists felt the need to be secretive or "closeted" about their sexual orientation. They described obstacles to obtaining a psychiatric residency by physicians known to be homosexual. They reviewed the well-known discriminatory policies of psychoanalytic institutes that considered lesbian and gay candidates unfit for training (Drescher, 1995; Isay, 1996; Magee and Miller, 1997).

Following the plenary session presentation, the discussion period began with a memorable 10 to 12 minutes of tense silence, an awkward reaction that seemed to mirror the anxiety, confusion, and conflict about homosexuality present in the psychiatric profession as a whole. The dialogue that followed was also more anxiety laden than usual, despite GAP's long history of focusing on controversial topics. It was productive, however, and in 1987 the Committee on Human Sexuality was established and chose as its first subject of study "Antihomosexual Bias in Psychiatry and Psychotherapy."

In this report, we identify and draw attention to the problem of bias against lesbians and gay men as it exists in psychiatry and the practice of psychotherapy. The manifestations of bias are seen in the treatment of patients and in the education and training of mental health professionals. We also discuss relevant presentations of antihomosexual bias (AHB) in the legal system, as well as in the general medical response to patients infected by the Human Immunodeficiency Virus (HIV) and those who have Acquired Immunodeficiency Syndrome (AIDS).

The Committee on Human Sexuality of the Group for the Advancement of Psychiatry chose this subject because of our increasing awareness of the harmful effects of AHB on patients and their therapists alike, on the progress of treatment and on the reputation of the mental health profession itself. The issue appears more and more often in daily practice, in teaching and supervision, and in the public press.

The members of the Committee on Human Sexuality of GAP are a diverse group of psychiatrists, coming from different social, clinical and theoretical backgrounds. While recognizing that our personal and professional histories have inevitably helped to shape our views, we have attempted to present a balanced description of the ways in which AHB affects the teaching and the practice of psychiatry.

Antihomosexual bias is widespread in many cultures, including our own. It is difficult to think of anyone in our society (including lesbians and gay men themselves) who is able to avoid its impact. Therefore, it should not be surprising that mental health professionals, as members of a society, also consciously and unconsciously absorb that society's values. When this bias is selectively inattended, it may operate outside of conscious awareness. It is not realistic to expect that recognition of a bias will automatically eliminate it. Prejudice of any kind is not easily modified or shed, even with the best motives. However, we hope to encourage practicing psychiatrists and psychotherapists to recognize when they are speaking with or acting on a bias that previously would have been outside their awareness. This will enable professionals in our field to be better able to prevent AHB from affecting treatment and to understand and assist their gay and lesbian patients.

Acknowledgments

This GAP Report, *Homosexuality and the Mental Health Professions: The Impact of Bias,"* has been a long time in the making, and the Committee on Human Sexuality, which produced it, has a large debt of gratitude to many persons that needs to be expressed.

Henry Work and Michael Zales were instrumental in helping to establish a Committee on Human Sexuality within the GAP framework, which opened the door to an examination of the issues that the present report addresses—not an easy task. The encouragement from Judd Marmor, a former president of GAP, was very influential in promoting the acceptance of the newly formed Committee. Martha Kirkpatrick and Harold Lief were most helpful as early advisors.

The original members of this Committee should be recognized for their courage in coming together to form this fledgling group, which was at first regarded with some skepticism by many GAP members. The founding members were the late John Spiegel and I, soon joined by Paul Adams, Peggy Hanley-Hackenbruck, Joan Lang, Stuart Nichols, and Terry Stein. Not long after, we were joined by Debbie Carter, Johanna Hoffman, and the late Harris Peck. This original group of individuals established a presence within GAP, providing greater visibility and a forum for open discussions of gay and lesbian issues, and they gave this report its initial momentum. I deeply regret that John Spiegel and Harris Peck did not live to see the completed report.

Early on, while searching for a research topic to address in a GAP report, the Committee hosted talks by three outside consultants: James Weinrich, Phyllis Chessler, and Tom Mazur. The discussions within the Committee that followed their presentations helped to clarify the future direction of the Committee's work.

For several years, the Committee worked arduously on the production of a potentially comprehensive handbook on homosexuality and psychiatry intended for medical students, psychiatric residents, practicing psychiatrists, psychologists, social workers, nurses, and the like. As time went on, the Committee became mired in the enormity of that task, and it gradually became clear that this noble goal was overly ambitious, given the limitations of GAP's traditional way of working in semiannual, two-day Committee meetings.

In order to reconceive and focus the Committee's efforts and to produce a publishable report in the near future, Richard C. Friedman and Jack Drescher, both well known for their expertise and writing skills, were asked to join the Committee. They were later followed by Joseph Merlino and Jennifer Downey. At the same time, Justin Richardson, in his capacity as a Ginsburg Fellow, made a vital contribution to the section of this monograph related to HIV and AIDS; Richard A. Friedman, a faculty member at Cornell Medical Center, provided valuable assistance as a consultant to the Committee. As a result of intense discussions, the Committee adopted the present report's emphasis on antihomosexual bias (AHB) in the mental health professions.

I wish to thank three other Ginsburg Fellows who participated in our Committee's work: Martha Bird; John Burton, who made many substantive and editorial contributions; and Gwen Zornberg, to whom we owe special gratitude, along with her associate, Pauline Quirion, for contributing the important chapter on the legal manifestations of antihomosexual bias.

Christina Sekaer, who attended Committee meetings as a guest, deserves special recognition for her brilliant observations and literary acumen. I look forward to her joining the Committee as a member.

As the report neared readiness for publication, Knight Aldrich reviewed it critically, line by line, and we are grateful for his trenchant observations on both its substance and its style. Carol Nadelson gave astute advice in her role as a member of the GAP Publications Committee. Frances Roton, Executive Director of GAP, has been a most supportive resource for the Committee.

This report could not have come to publication without Jack Drescher, currently Chair of the Committee on Human Sexuality. When the initial publishers ran into difficulties getting the report to press, it was he who resourcefully contacted The Analytic Press and later took charge of the final complex editing process. Jack's forceful leadership saved the day and made this report a reality.

My deep personal thanks go to Mark Koenig, who was my secretary during much of the time that this report was being prepared. He spent long hours editing, copying, and mailing out the many manuscript versions that were required during the period of my Chairmanship of the Committee on Human Sexuality, from 1987 to the completion of the report in November 1998.

Bertram Schaffner, MD
New York City
November 21, 1999

This GAP Report was long in the making, and at this juncture it must be noted that it owes its very existence to the ongoing perseverance and dedication of one man: Bertram Schaffner, M.D. The members of the Committee on Human Sexuality know Bert well and are keenly aware of his great modesty. Because of his unwillingness to draw attention to himself, those who do not know him well are unaware of his many professional accomplishments throughout this last half century. Bert has done much to enrich the professional lives of his professional colleagues and the personal lives of his friends and patients. He has singularly done more on a personal basis for gay psychiatrists and psychotherapists than any other figure known to us.

Bert took on a challenge as founding Chair of the GAP Committee on Human Sexuality and did so at a time of his life when most people have already gone into retirement. Even today, Bert is working full time. Even overtime. His capacity for finding pleasure in his work has been an inspiration to many. Bert works diligently, patiently, cautiously when he can, expeditiously when necessary, and always thoughtfully. But, above all, Bert works.

Bert has provided what Winnicott called a "holding environment" for a number of high-risk professional endeavors, this monograph on antihomosexual bias being just the latest. As most GAP members know, writing an article by committee, let alone a monograph of this magnitude, is an almost impossible venture. Furthermore, GAP's Committee on Human Sexuality comprises members with strong personalities and disparate views of what should be the report's primary focus. Bert's gift was to allow the individual group members' creative differences to emerge while keeping the Committee focused on a difficult, common task. A few eggs were broken in the making of this omelet. However, this monograph illustrates what a successful "chef" Bert has been. For that, and for so much more, Bert has earned the deepest respect of the members of the Committee on Human Sexuality, who dedicate this monograph to him.

Committee on Human Sexuality
Group for the Advancement of Psychiatry
White Plains, New York
November 21, 1999

1 DIMENSIONS OF ANTIHOMOSEXUAL BIAS

Historical Influences on AHB

Negative perceptions of homosexuality are rooted in many aspects of our history and culture. These include:

1. *Biblical interpretation:* From early in the history of Judeo Christian cultures, there has been a tendency to condemn homosexual behavior, by emphasizing Biblical admonitions against it (Genesis 19, Leviticus 18: 7,22, Leviticus 20:13, Judges 19, I Kings 22:46, II Kings 23:7, Romans 1:27, I Corinthians 6:9, I Timothy 1:9-10).

2. *Sin to illness:* The scientific and medical construction of a category representing a particular social group, the term homosexual was coined in the 19th century. Its rapid and widespread usage by the public, as well as by the medical profession, reflected an attempt to replace religious,

condemning explanations with more compassionate, scientific ones. The homosexual/heterosexual binary obscured the variety of ways in which one could characterize sexual or other conduct (Bullough, 1979; Gonsiorek, 1991).

3. *Degeneracy theory:* Influential in Europe and the United States in the 19th century, degeneracy theory proposed that traits associated with undesirable social behaviors were inherited. According to this theory, homosexuality, like violent criminality, enuresis, and alcoholism, was seen as manifestations of hereditary degeneracy. Thus, this was an early biological theory of homosexuality. Degeneracy theory also illustrated how the concepts of vice and illness are often interchangeable (Krafft-Ebing, 1886; Walter, 1956; Foucault, 1978; Greenberg, 1988).

4. *Antisexual Victorianism:* In the 19th century, the Victorian culture's repressive stance toward sexual pleasure was expressed in diverse ways, including the widespread belief that masturbation caused insanity or could lead to homosexuality (Acton, 1865; Rosenthal, 1985; Duberman, 1986, 1991). Victorian sensibility also nourished the concepts of contagion and quarantine, beliefs that both fostered and were derived from degeneracy theories. It was popularly believed, for example, that homosexuality could be transmitted by sexually active people and that people who otherwise would develop as heterosexuals could be "corrupted" by mutual masturbation with a person of the same sex (Bullough, 1979; Weeks, 1985).

5. *Idealization of the nuclear family:* Social philosophers of the 18th and 19th centuries emphasized the intimate link between the health of society as a whole and the stability of the nuclear family organized around traditional sex roles. The so-called traditional family became a symbol not only of social cohesion and economic stability, but of correct moral behavior as well. This belief contributed to the development of a heterosexist ethic (Greenberg, 1988).

6. *Heterosexism:* Heterosexism is a belief in the inherent superiority of social practices and cultural institutions associated with heterosexuality, such as monogamy, marriage, and child rearing in two-parent, heterosexual families. In its more benign form, it might be referred to as "heterocentrism." In its more malignant presentations, heterosexism is the ideological system that denies, denigrates, and stigmatizes any nonheterosexual form of behavior, identity, relationship, or community (Greenberg, 1988; Herek, 1990, 1995).

Attitudes Toward Homosexuality

Attitudes in the General Population

There is a dearth of articles in the psychiatric literature on attitudes toward homosexuality in the general population. We hope to stimulate further research in this area.

An important national survey of sexual morality and experience was carried out under the auspices of the Institute for Sex Research at Indiana University in 1970 (Klassen, Williams, and Levitt, 1989). With the help of the National Opinion Research Center, the investigators obtained a representative national sample of more than 3,000 men and women. Interviews revealed that 60% of these individuals believed that lesbians and gay men have unusually strong sex drives and that those who are older commonly seduce younger ones who, as a consequence, then become homosexual. Seventy per cent were concerned that lesbians and gay men seek to become sexually involved with children; half the 70% strongly believed this to be the case. The fear that lesbians and gay men constitute a threat to children was substantial even among the subgroup of the sample whose overall attitudes toward homosexuality were not particularly negative. More than two-thirds of the sample felt that lesbians and gay men should be barred from teaching, the ministry, the judiciary, medical practice, and government service. Almost 50% believed that homosexuality can cause the downfall of civilization. In this investigation, the most powerful predictor of attitudes toward homosexuality was the intensity of religious belief. People with these attitudes were more likely to come from the deep South or Midwest and from religious families that tended to be sexually repressive. A subsequent study by Nyberg and Alston (1977), of a representative sample of more than 1,000 white American adults, found that over 72% believed that homosexual relations were "always wrong."

With the passage of time, public opinion has become more accepting and tolerant. For example, a Gallup poll in 1989 revealed that 71% of respondents believed that gay men and women should have equal job opportunities (Colasanto, 1989). The reasons for this shift in public opinion are not entirely clear. Certainly, the emergence of articulate gay and lesbian spokespeople may be a factor. The AIDS epidemic may have played a role as well. According to polls, the public perception of a minority group struggling valiantly with a dread disease led to the diminution of prejudice and discrimination in some quarters.

The equating of AIDS with homosexuality, however, has also led to an escalation of fearful and hateful attitudes toward gay men and, ironically, to lesbians. Reports of escalating violence against people perceived to be gay suggest that opinion polls do not fully measure the extent of antihomosexual attitudes in the general population. The reported incidence of violence against gay and lesbian persons is increasing in many major American cities and appears to be increasing more rapidly than other bias-related crimes, such as racially motivated hate crimes. Major problems with antigay and lesbian violence and harassment have been reported at college and university campuses, including Yale, Rutgers, Penn State, the University of Massachusetts at Amherst, the University of Illinois at Champaign-Urbana, and other sites. At Yale, of 166 gay and lesbian students studied, 24% had been threatened, 24% followed or chased, and 5% beaten. Fifty-seven per cent reported that they feared for their safety. At the high school and junior high school levels as well, antigay and antilesbian violence and harassment are widespread (Cort and Corlevale, 1982; Herek and Berrill, 1992; Klinger and Stein 1996). Teenagers surveyed about bias responded more negatively to gay people than to other minorities.

In a review of research on those holding negative attitudes toward lesbians and gay men, Herek (1984) found several similarities among diverse samples. When compared with those with more favorable attitudes toward lesbians and gay men, people with AHB were less likely to a) have had known personal contact with lesbians or gay men; and b) report having engaged in homosexual behavior or to identify themselves as lesbian or gay.

They were also more likely to c) perceive their peers as manifesting negative attitudes toward gay people, especially when the respondents are males; d) have lived in areas where intolerance of homosexuality is more the norm (e.g., the Midwestern and Southern United States, the Canadian prairies, and in rural areas or small towns), especially during adolescence; e) be older and less educated; f) be devoutly religious, attend church frequently, subscribe to a conservative religious philosophy; g) express traditional, restrictive attitudes about sex roles; h) manifest guilt or negativity about sexuality and to be less permissive sexually; and i) manifest high levels of authoritarianism and related personality characteristics.

Herek noted that negative attitudes may serve different functions for a person and that people may share similar attitudes for different reasons:

> First, such attitudes may be *experiential*, categorizing social reality primarily on the basis of one's past interactions with lesbian and gay people. Second, attitudes may be mainly *defensive*, helping a person to cope with some inner conflicts or anxiety by projecting it onto gay men and lesbians. Finally, attitudes may be *symbolic*, expressing abstract ideological concepts that are closely linked to one's own notion of self and to one's social networks and reference groups [p. 8].

In general, men manifest more negative attitudes toward gay people than do women. Violence against lesbian and gay victims is usually perpetrated by males, as is true of violence in general (Moyer, 1974; Herek and Berrill, 1992). Heterosexually identified men and women alike tend to have more negative attitudes toward people of their own gender who are perceived to be lesbian and gay than toward people of the other gender (San Miguel and Millham, 1976). There are no studies of the profiles of mental health professionals or how likely they are to share some of the culture's stereotypical beliefs about lesbian and gay people.

Attitudes Within Dynamic Psychiatry

Persistent AHB is often rooted more in personal value systems and experiences than in the scientific literature. Since bias is often rationalized or denied, its effects may be especially pervasive and debilitating. An example of a common rationalization of bias is that a homosexual orientation is intrinsically more pathological than a heterosexual one. This kind of rationalization may lead to discrimination against patients and trainees.

During the years after World War II until the 1970s, American psychiatry's formulations of homosexuality were largely based on psychoanalytic models and common cultural stereotypes of human behavior (Lewes, 1988). In the *American Psychiatric Association's Diagnostic and Statistical Manual*, first edition (DSM-I: American Psychiatric Association, 1952), homosexuality was classified as a sociopathic personality disorder (Bayer, 1981). In the DSM-II (American Psychiatric Association, 1968), it was reclassified as a sexual deviation. The DSM-II was revised in 1973 and homosexuality per se was removed as a diagnostic category (Bayer, 1981).

The pathologizing psychoanalytic theories of homosexuality, as well as the interactive influence of theory and culture, are too extensive to be discussed more than briefly here. The reader interested in these areas is referred to Bieber et al.

(1962), Weideman (1962, 1974), Socarides (1968, 1978), Ruitenbeek (1963), Sulloway (1979), Marmor (1980), Bayer (1981), Fisher and Greenberg (1985), Gay (1988), Greenberg (1988), Isay (1989), Lewes (1988), Friedman (1988), Holt (1989), O'Connor and Ryan (1993), Mitchell (1996), Magee and Miller (1997), and Drescher (1998b).

During the socially conservative years following World War II, policy positions taken regarding homosexuality by such institutions as the military and the law were buttressed by pathologizing psychoanalytic constructs. Lewes (1988) has pointed out that, during that era, many psychoanalysts couched their own personal endorsement of traditional religious and family values in supposedly objective psychoanalytic terminology. The image of psychological health was defined as a nuclear family organized around traditional gender roles (Bieber et al., 1962).

The psychiatric literature underemphasized and ignored lesbian and gay people whose capacities to love and work were unimpaired (Hooker, 1957). It also ignored the negative countertransference toward these patients (Mitchell, 1978, 1981; Kwawer, 1980; Lewes, 1988; Frommer, 1995) and the influence of widespread social prejudice on their psychological well-being (Stein and Cohen, 1986; Isay, 1989; Drescher, 1998b).

The psychodynamic literature of that era focused on the etiology of homosexuality, which was presumed to result primarily from preoedipal or oedipal psychic trauma, in contrast to heterosexuality which was assumed to unfold naturally and which therefore had no "etiology" (Bergler, 1944, 1951, 1956; Bieber et al., 1962; Socarides, 1968; Bayer, 1981). Homosexuality was believed to be a sign of psychosexual immaturity. Any role of neurobiological influences on sexual orientation was deemphasized and even denigrated in favor of psychodynamic hypotheses (Lewes, 1988; Friedman and Downey, 1993a, b).

After the American Psychiatric Association removed the diagnosis of homosexuality from its list of mental disorders in 1973, other organizations of mental health professionals soon reached similar conclusions. These groups included the American Psychological Association and the National Association of Social Workers. A careful review of scientific evidence indicated that there was no clear-cut, demonstrable relationship between sexual orientation and psychopathological symptoms or disorders.

The original decision by the American Psychiatric Association to remove homosexuality from the category of pathology was opposed by a substantial minority of psychiatrists (Bayer, 1981). Subsequently, however, a 1977 survey of 2,500 psychiatrists found that a majority felt that homosexuality is pathological and that lesbians and gay men are less capable than heterosexuals of mature, loving relationships (Lief, 1977). Studies of other mental health professionals found that many, sometimes a majority, have had negative attitudes about homosexuality and lesbian and gay people and continue to harbor them (Fort et al., 1971; Clark, 1975; Rudolph, 1989, 1990; Lilling and Friedman, 1995; Friedman and Lilling, 1996).

Until recently there was a notable absence of openly lesbian and gay psychoanalysts willing to criticize the inadequacy of the prevailing psychoanalytic theoretical models of sexual orientation. Although some gay and lesbian psychiatrists began speaking openly and critically of psychoanalytic theory in the mid-1980s, it was not until the 1990s that gay-identified psychoanalysts began to write or speak against prevailing models on the basis of their personal and clinical experience (Blechner, 1993; O'Connor and Ryan, 1993; Domenici and Lesser, 1995; Isay, 1996; Drescher, 1997, 1998b; Magee and Miller, 1997). Thus, an important data source was not available for decades. These new contributions can be analogized to the ways in which women mental health professionals challenged earlier, prevailing phallocentric theories (Lewes, 1988). The appearance of increasing numbers of openly gay and lesbian psychotherapists within mainstream psychiatric organizations suggests that heterosexual psychoanalytic attitudes are being challenged and may even have undergone substantial changes.

Research scientists have accumulated substantial data indicating that homosexuality per se is not associated with psychopathology any more than is heterosexuality. In any event, personality measures, projective tests, rates of psychiatric symptoms, and lifetime prevalence of psychiatric disorders, with few exceptions, do not distinguish between homosexual and heterosexual subjects (Gonsiorek and Weinrich, 1991; Friedman and Downey, 1994; Cabaj and Stein, 1996). Two types of psychological difficulties have been reported to be more frequent in lesbian and gay populations: attempted (but not completed) suicide in youth (Robins, 1981; Rich et al., 1986; Hendin, 1992; Prenzlauer, Drescher, and Winchel, 1992; Schafer, 1995) and substance abuse (Friedman and Downey, 1994). Even these findings await replication, however, and are not conclusive. Furthermore, studies have corroborated the role that stress plays in the lives of lesbians and gay men and the impact it has on their mental health. Increased exposure to stress might explain why the lifetime history of depression is elevated in gay men, although present history of depression is not (Williams et al., 1991).

Overall, psychodynamic psychiatry in the 1990s has discarded the paradigm that homosexuality is inherently pathological and has adopted the normal variant model. Psychodynamic psychiatric clinicians currently recognize that gay and lesbian patients usually seek treatment for the same reasons that heterosexual patients do: Axis I and Axis II psychiatric disorders, and stress, leading to suffering and disability. The full impact of these changes within psychiatry on future social, medical, legal, religious, and political institutions remains to be seen.

Attitudes in Fundamentalist Religion

Religious fundamentalists have expressed disparaging views about lesbians and gay men. Some have rationalized and others exhorted violence in their public rhetoric. For example, "When civil legislation is introduced to protect behavior to which no one has any conceivable right, neither the Church nor society at large should be surprised when other distorted notions and practices gain ground, and irrational and violent reactions increase" (Congregation for the Doctrine of the Faith, 1986, paragraph 10, in Herek and Berrill, 1992, pp. 90–91). Many conservative religious groups and movements depict lesbian and gay people as being profligate and immoral and attribute the AIDS epidemic to punishment for sexual "sins." The category "homosexual" has become, in the minds of many, a symbol of one who rejects all of society's rules. From this perspective, homosexual practices must be violently resisted, or else abuse and neglect of traditional family values and structures will inevitably follow.

Conservative mental health professionals appear to subscribe to similar views. So, for example, in a famous case in which a gay man was murdered after revealing his attraction to a heterosexual neighbor, one well-known psychoanalyst blamed "the gay rights movement for the Jenny Jones incident.... To turn the world upside down and say it doesn't matter if we are homosexual or heterosexual is folly ... to ask for total acceptance and enthusiastic approval of homosexuality as a normal and valuable psychosexual institution is truly tempting social and personal disaster" (Socarides, quoted in Dunlap, 1995).

Definitions and Issues

The term homosexuality refers to an erotic attraction to persons of the same anatomical gender; bisexuality, to attraction to persons of both sexes; and heterosexuality, to attraction to persons of the other sex. While the terms may suggest categorical divisions between types of sexual orientation, in fact attraction is usefully conceptualized as existing along a continuum. People experience either extremes of same or other sex attraction on the continuum, and others experience some degree of attraction to both sexes (Kinsey, Pomeroy, and

Martin, 1948; Money, 1988). By erotic attraction, we mean that the person experiences the psychophysiological changes of sexual arousal with imagery of males, females, or both. We use the term sexual orientation instead of sexual preference because orientation denotes only direction of attraction, not motivation or conscious choice. Sexual preference suggests willful decision making as to the objects of erotic desire. As a general rule, homosexual, bisexual, and heterosexual orientation are not consciously experienced as volitional processes (Friedman, 1988; Isay, 1989; Money, 1989). Sexual activity, on the other hand, is frequently volitional. Thus, there are often incongruities between desire/arousal and behavior.

Many, but not all, persons who are predominantly or exclusively homosexual in their sexual orientation are referred to in this monograph as gay or lesbian. Gay or lesbian connotes an awareness of one's homosexual orientation and often an involvement in social and political communities of other individuals with similar sexual orientation. Thus, persons who may be primarily homosexual in their sexual attraction may not necessarily view themselves, nor be viewed, as gay or lesbian unless they also acknowledge and are accepting of their sexual orientation, affiliate with other persons who share this orientation in some manner, and assume some aspects of personal identity associated with their homosexuality. Furthermore, in this report, the word homosexual is not used as a noun (e.g., "He is a homosexual"), but rather as an adjective (e.g., homosexual attraction). Usage as a noun takes sexual orientation, one aspect of a person, and reifies that singular characteristic to label the whole person, often in a stigmatizing, prejudicial fashion (Magee and Miller, 1995, 1997).

Identity as gay, lesbian, or bisexual can be seen as a facet of what Erik Erikson (1959) termed ego identity. This psychological construct refers to identification with a group's attitudes and values and to a continuing sense of self-cohesion over time. Ego identity is formed during adolescence. When it is intact, the person is able to function autonomously, with a sense of uniqueness, while feeling connected to others. Some consider themselves gay but experience erotic arousal to stimuli of both sexes. They place more weight on the homoerotic than on the heteroerotic component for their sense of identity. Others with similar histories of erotic arousal consider themselves heterosexual, and still others label themselves bisexual. Ego identity should not be confused with gender identity, which refers to the enduring awareness that one is either male or female. Because he believed this awareness is a fundamental component of the self-image of most people, the psychoanalyst Robert Stoller (1968) labeled it core gender identity. It is now thought that one's core gender identity is synthesized as the result of complex social, biological, and psychological influences. Social learning, physiological predisposition, and cognitive factors interact to lead a child to label herself or himself as "I am female" or "I am male." Studies of intersexed persons, patients with psychiatric disorders, and normal children suggest that core gender identity is usually formed by the third year of life.

Gender role behaviors are social enactments. They consist of the things one says and does that advertise one's gender identity to others (Money and Ehrhardt, 1972). Concepts of masculinity and femininity may vary in differing social contexts, whereas the ongoing self-assessment of one's masculine and feminine performance, the core gender identity, may endure as a permanent trait.

The term gender identity differentiation was originally invoked by Money to indicate the similarity between the psychological processes involved in establishment of core gender identity and those involved in cellular differentiation. It suggests that the early childhood process of gender identity differentiation is best conceptualized as a continuation of embryologically occurring sexual differentiation of the central nervous and reproductive systems.

Ego identity is formed much later, during adolescence and young adulthood. Core gender identity can be thought of as a component of ego identity in the same way that one's native language is part of one's identity. The field of gender identity studies is relatively new, having emerged long after original theories about sexual orientation put forth by Freud (1905, 1910, 1920, 1933, 1937) and others (Krafft-Ebing, 1886; Ellis, 1938) had exerted great influence on clinical theorizing. Contemporary clinicians need to be consistently aware of the distinction between gender identity and ego identity.

The difference between gender identity and sexual orientation is an important concept. This distinction was frequently blurred in the clinical literature pertaining to homosexuality, particularly during the three decades immediately following World War II (Friedman, 1988). Thus, passivity, effeminacy, and homosexuality were frequently conflated in discussions about gay men, while activity, masculinity, and homosexuality were the nouns used in discussions about lesbians (Freud, 1905; Bergler, 1944, 1951, 1956; Socarides, 1968; Bayer, 1981).

Homophobia has been given a variety of meanings and has been used in vague, nonspecific ways. The term originally referred to fear of gay persons or of homosexuality itself (Weinberg, 1972) but has grown to include any antigay or antilesbian belief, feeling, or behavior. Heterosexism, which we defined earlier, is sometimes used as a synonym for Weinberg's original description of external homophobia. Weinberg also defined the category of internalized homophobia as the self-hatred that many lesbians and gay men experience toward their own homosexual identities, attractions, and world. The origins of homophobia lie in both societal and individual factors (Herek, 1984). Many expressions of homophobia represent accepted views of gender and sexual norms in our own society and others. For example, homosexuality continues to be condemned by many institutions, particularly religious and military groups (Jones and Koshes, 1995), in spite of the damaging effects of such prejudices on both gay and lesbian persons and on the institutions themselves. Prejudicial associations of homosexuality with gender nonconformity is still used to enforce gender role conformity. This is done by social condemnation of effeminate behavior in boys and men, and of masculine behavior in girls and women, under the assumption that these behaviors are synonymous with homosexuality. The deleterious effects of socially condoned homophobia are manifested in the outbreaks of antigay and antilesbian violence, demands for the limitation of civil rights of gay persons, and its damaging effects on the psychological well-being of gays and lesbians who experience discrimination and stigmatization.

Homophobia is particularly destructive at an individual level when it occurs within the context of a psychotherapeutic relationship (Moss, 1992, 1997). In this report, we examine the ways that this prejudice is often expressed in psychotherapy and its distressing effects on patients, the course of therapy, and their therapists. We use the term antihomosexual bias (AHB) rather than homophobia since the former seems more specific and better describes the phenomena we are discussing.

Psychological Mechanisms in AHB

Paranoid Mechanisms

Classical psychoanalytic theory defined paranoia as a defense against unconcious homosexual wishes (Freud, 1911). Few clinicians today would explain paranoia on the basis of repressed homosexuality. There does, however, seem to be a clinical correlation between some forms of antihomosexual feelings and paranoid phenomena. Numerous psychodynamic pathways can lead to negative attitudes toward people perceived to be homosexual.

Paranoid psychodynamics occur along a spectrum of severity from persons with paranoid tendencies who are otherwise functional to psychotic, delusional patients. Some people function well but have a tendency to look at the world through an internal filter that is referential, suspicious, and mistrustful. In some people, this paranoid tendency is state related, while in some it appears to reflect a dominant personality style. Paranoid psychodynamics involve a sense of perceived threat not only to the self, but to the gender identity of the self. A man under the influence of such dynamics tends to experience a solid sense of core gender identity—he knows he is male—but has insecurity about his feelings of masculinity. This psychodynamic component is similar to that experienced by most boys (see AHB in Boys). What is different, however, is the intense anger and anxiety triggered by the sense of gender/self vulnerability in these men. Rageful affect, coupled with cognitive distortions stemming from the use of projection, leads to the belief that the man is the innocent victim of malevolence expressed toward him by others. He therefore feels justified in defending himself in a hostile environment by attacking his "enemies" (Friedman, 1988).

The gender insecurity of paranoid men who are also psychotic often leads them to experience delusions and hallucinations with homosexual content (Klein and Horowitz, 1949; Klaf and Davis, 1960; Planansky and Johnston, 1962). These men equate being unmasculine with being homosexual. Interestingly, psychotic paranoid women do not tend to experience homosexual delusions. Instead, they experience delusions (and hallucinations) with disparaging heterosexual content, for example, "slut, whore, cunt." One psychodynamic explanation could be that the loss of self-integrity associated with paranoid psychoses is experienced by men and women as penetration of the body, represented as oral or anal penetration by men and vaginal penetration by women. A feminist interpretation would be that the gay-disparaged man and the slut-disparaged woman are both being maligned as women. In a society with a double standard, a "fag" is denigrated but a "Don Juan" is admired.

The paranoid psychodynamics of delusional or hallucinating patients may reveal, in amplified form, some psychological mechanisms found among people engaging in violent AHB. Although data about nonpsychotic violent persons are sparse, clinical experience suggests that they are probably people who are easily humiliated and who respond to the demands of intimate relationships or competitive defeat and loss of power and stature with emergency emotional states (Sullivan, 1953, 1956; Cameron, 1967; Ovesey, 1969). The sense of painful humiliation generates the need to scapegoat others, particularly "homosexuals," who become the repository of projected negative attributes.

Phobic Mechanisms

Homophobia, as a simple phobia, appears to be quite rare, although there are no data indicating its actual prevalence within the general or clinical population. For this reason we prefer the term antihomosexual bias or AHB. However, phobic mechanisms probably operate in some people who express AHB. In these people, defense mechanisms of repression, projection, displacement, and avoidance lead to a consciously experienced irrational fear. The dreaded object is avoided, thus allowing the phobic person to function without having to experience key conflicts from within. The specific object that symbolically represents conflicts that the phobic person seeks to avoid may be chosen as a consequence of actual experiences the person had with similar objects during childhood (Fenichel, 1945). Perhaps some people with phobic predispositions during childhood had experiences that endowed homosexuality with a unique, personal valence, allowing it to be selected as a phobic symbol later in life. Others may be phobic/avoidant toward sexuality in general and displace this avoidance onto homosexuality.

Phobias may also arise in people with obsessional character structures. Here, the avoided stimulus often symbolizes loss of control of aggressivity. An obsessional person who is angry at his boss, for example, may as a consequence of isolation of affect, experience an intrusive, ego-alien repetitive thought, "Shoot your boss." He may then phobically avoid guns and places where guns are sold or used. The reasons that obsessional people may develop phobias of homosexuality are diverse and a function of the different meaning that homosexuality has in the personal scripts of such people. Classical psychoanalytic theory has stated that obsessional people often ascribe special meaning to anality, and it is possible that the image of anal sexuality becomes a phobic stimulus in some cases (Fenichel, 1945). In any event, much research needs to be done in this area.

Internalized Homophobia

Given our culture's profound endorsement of heterosexuality, it is understandable that children who grow up to become gay or lesbian experience difficulties with self-esteem as adults (Cabaj and Stein, 1996). There is a tendency for a stigmatized person to internalize a damaged or "spoiled" identity (Goffman, 1963). Thus, many patients come to loathe themselves for being "homosexual." The specific meaning of antihomosexual attitudes will vary from person to person. These attitudes in lesbians and gay men may result from identification with covert or overt parental attitudes regarding masculinity, femininity, and homosexuality. Antihomosexual attitudes may be internalized as a consequence of painful childhood interactions with peers (Downey and Friedman, 1995b, 1996; Friedman and Downey, 1995; Drescher, 1998b).

Most gay and lesbian patients have found it necessary to hide their inner lives from others for prolonged periods of time. Sometimes, particularly during their early years, these patients may be so influenced by the heterosexually oriented culture in which they are raised that they successfully deny the significance of their own erotic fantasies. Such patients learn to adopt heterosocial mannerisms and behaviors, as actors learn to assume the roles of characters in a play. Sometimes they believe that by so doing they will influence their erotic fantasies to become heterosexual like those of their peers. Whether or not homosexual desires are denied, they are usually hidden from others at first. Young people often realize that their families and friends might well reject them were they to reveal their homosexual orientation. Conflicts about disclosure of sexual orientation are a commonly occurring cause of depression in gay and lesbian patients, particularly during adolescence and young adulthood, with distressing numbers of suicides and suicide attempts (Cabaj and Stein, 1996). The psychodynamic consequences of the necessity to live a double life because of prejudice and discrimination are just beginning to be systematically described. While the term "coming out" has become part of popular culture, psychiatrists and other mental health providers need to be educated to understand the multitudinous ramifications of this process. For example, some people may become aware of their same-sex feelings only in middle or late life. Gay men and lesbians need to constantly assess the impact that revealing their sexuality might have in their ongoing daily activities.

Internalized homophobia is organized around shame, guilt, anger, anxiety, and loneliness. Its many manifestations depend on the degree to which the representational world of the person is integrated or fragmented and the type of character defenses he or she uses. Among its major adverse consequences are vocational or educational underachievement; a sense of lack of entitlement to give and receive love, resulting in irrational efforts to undermine love relationships; and projection of a devalued self-image to a partner who is then scapegoated. Unconscious antihomosexual attitudes are so common among gay and lesbian patients that some therapists believe they are universal. To achieve a positive and psychologically well-adjusted identity, a person needs to be able to minimize the effects of AHB by challenging and neutralizing the denigrating assumptions of heterosexism and coming to value and affirm his or her homosexuality instead. It is important to note that, in spite of these impediments and challenges, many persons, with or without the help of therapy, have managed to overcome internalized and societal AHB and achieve lives rich in work, love, and play. This achievement may be more common today as public attitudes toward homosexuality become somewhat more tolerant and accepting. Studies that show how people successfully adapt to their own internalized homophobia provide an area of future research.

The Impact of AHB on Psychological Growth and Development

Although definitive studies are lacking, a psychodynamic developmental frame of reference can help us to conceptualize some of the origins of antihomosexual bias.

There is widespread cultural confusion between what are referred to as gender identity and sexual orientation. Thus, insecurity about one's own gender role may raise questions about one's sexual orientation and may sometimes contribute to an irrational fear of homosexuality. These fears may often underlie strongly negative attitudes and beliefs about gay or lesbian persons. Security about one's own gender role and sexual orientation appears to protect against fear of homosexuality.

AHB in Boys

Both gender insecurity and intolerance of homosexuality appear to be more problematic in men than in women. Some explanation for this difference may lie in gender-specific developmental psychodynamics. Many authors believe that a man's sense of masculinity appears to be a more vulnerable psychological achievement than a woman's sense of her femininity (Greenson, 1968; Stoller, 1974). Gilligan (1982) and Chodorow (1978) offer developmental theories that might explain this difference. They suggest that, because the primary caretaker for all children is almost universally a female, there are profound consequences for the way that boys and girls experience feelings of attachment and gender-valued self-esteem. For females, interpersonal intimacy may become associated with a sense of strengthened gender security and self-regard. Boys, however, develop their gender identity in the context of separating from the mother. According to Gilligan (1982), masculinity is defined through separation while femininity is defined through attachment. She further contends that male gender identity is threatened by intimacy while female gender identity is threatened by separation.

Psychoanalysts Greenson (1968) and Stoller (1974) have pointed out that there is a tendency in all children to identify with their primary caretaker. Boys must develop a masculine identity against the gradient of motivations arising from maternal identifications. Although most boys appear able to accomplish the developmental task of disidentification, they may always need to defend against the "pull" of their original feminine identifications. (Discussing reasons that this defensive need occurs more in some children than in others is beyond the scope of this report.)

The relationship between masculine self-esteem and antihomosexual attitudes is particularly important between ages six and twelve. This is illustrated in an investigation of preadolescent baseball players carried out by Fine (1987), who studied the behavior of boys on 10 Little League teams in Massachusetts and Minnesota. Fine was mindful that adult sex roles are formed in childhood. He found that Little Leaguers are highly moral, that is, concerned with behaving in specific ways compatible with their values. Their moral universe is, however, quite different from the one that adults usually perceive. The peer group of these 11- and 12-year-old boys prescribed values that in adult life would be viewed as something of a parody of machismo. Toughness, courage, and control of emotional display were prized. Heterosexuality was positively sanctioned, but not deep emotional involvement with girls, which was likely to be seen as feminine overinvolvement. As far as homosexuality goes, Fine comments:

> Most of these boys have not met anyone who they believe "really" is a homosexual, and most of these boys do not know how to define homosexual other than to say they are boys who "like other boys" or "a guy who wants to marry another guy." Despite this, homosexuality was a central theme in their speech: "You're a faggot"; "God, he's gay"; "He's the biggest fag in the world"; "He sucks"; "What a queer"; "Kiss my ass" [p. 104].

In the world of these boys gentleness and nonassertiveness were equated with weakness and effeminacy, although none of the boys on the receiving end of insults were feminine in mannerism. Fine suggests that boys constantly feel the need to differentiate themselves from those who are female, weaker, and younger. That cursing and contemptuous scapegoating of peers were heavily organized around homosexual imagery suggests that such imagery reflects a central dimension of the way in which nonhomosexual American youths organize their thoughts about sex and violence. The boys on the teams studied in this investigation were not unusually cruel and, indeed, seemed to have many of the attributes expected in a sample of "normal" American children. The need to be accepted by peers, and particularly to be respected as masculine by male peers, often precedes adolescence and is a hallmark of the latency-age phase of development. The clinical literature dealing with problems of boys in this phase has tended to focus on the so-called sissies, rather than on the bullies in these encounters.

Adult attitudes and beliefs seem to be on a continuum with those of childhood, as is illustrated by the widespread derision expressed by men toward others who are perceived as being somehow not "masculine." Contempt, expressed in the term fag, for example, permeates the fabric of American mass culture. The term has multiple origins, all with a denigrating or demeaning dictionary context: according to the *Oxford English Dictionary*, "in English schools, a junior student performing tasks for a senior, a flap on a coat, a parasitic insect that infects sheep, a short form of 'faggot'—a bundle of twigs bound together for use as fuel, sometimes with the express purpose of burning heretics alive, or a term used to refer to women in a contemptuous manner." Evidence of adult attitudes may readily be found in popular movies, books, songs, and television and radio shows.

From the developmental, psychodynamic point of view, the sense of masculinity of many males is relatively fragile, at least from the latency-age phase of development, and may remain so throughout life. Scapegoating of persons labeled homosexual is a common mechanism by which such men with fragile identities, either as juveniles or adults, seek to cope with their insecurity about their own masculinity. Scapegoating serves the function of distancing the abuser from and feeling superior to the abused. A sense of masculine self-esteem can also be transiently bolstered by a feeling of power associated with the fantasy of dominating another male.

Boys tend to be negatively disposed toward those who are labeled "sissies", "fags", and "homosexuals." They do not appear to hold comparably negative perceptions of lesbians. In the minds of most juvenile boys, and probably many men as well, "homosexual" refers to males only.

AHB in Girls

Cross-gender role behavior in girls is generally much better tolerated by parents and other adults than it is in boys, especially before puberty. Girls also seem less threatened than boys by peers who do not conform to traditional gender-role stereotypes. On the other hand, epidemiological studies indicate that a considerable number of American women have negative attitudes toward both male and female homosexuality.

The issues of development of gender identity and sexual orientation in lesbians differ from those of gay men, although both groups must contend with the heterosexist values of our society. In fact, the differing attitudes toward male and female homosexuality are a lens through which one can see and understand the cultural valuing of masculinity and femininity. Boys who are called "fags" are being denigrated as being like girls—a gender slur—but they are also being called "girls", that is, members of the less valued sex in our heterosexist society. Tomboys are tolerated because they aspire to masculine values. Girls who are called tomboy are being denigrated as being like boys, a gender slur, but are actually being praised to the degree that they achieve masculine goals (such as beating the boys in baseball). Clinically, adult women patients may recall with pride having been "quite a tomboy" in their youth, whereas men invariably experience great hurt and shame in recalling having been labelled sissies. A further complication in comparing antihomosexual teasing of boys with antihomosexual teasing of girls relates to another factor in our society, the invisibility of lesbians. Women are traditionally seen as less sexual than men. Lesbian sexuality has been overlooked historically in many laws regulating gay male sexuality. Children's teasing may include "fag" more than "lezzy" because of a much stronger cultural awareness of gay men and the relative invisibility of lesbians. The counterpart to macho posturing in boys is the phenomenon of heterosexual teenage girls', insecure in their gender identity, adopting stereotypic female roles or even getting pregnant as ways to reinforce their sense of femaleness. That men are expected to be more sexual than women in our society affects women and lesbians in ways that are beyond the scope of this report.

Conclusions

Antihomosexual bias in the United States is part of a cultural tradition that traces its roots to aspects of the Judeo-Christian tradition (Moberly, 1983; Harvey, 1987). Nonetheless, scholars have pointed out that some aspects of that tradition have been accepting of homosexuality (Boswell, 1980, 1984; Pronk, 1993; Helminiak, 1994; Gomes, 1996). Among mental health professionals, the normal variant model of homosexuality is a relatively modern one and has proved sufficiently compelling to become the dominant clinical paradigm (Kinsey et al., 1948, 1953; Ford and Beach, 1951; Hooker, 1957; Bayer, 1981; DeCecco and Parker, 1995). Nevertheless, AHB is common in the culture at large and has an impact on the way clincians, patients, and families regard homosexuality. This chapter has discussed some of the historical beliefs that perpetuate AHB and has illustrated their impact on psychodynamic theory, modern religious fundamentalism, and the general population. The ubiquity of AHB has an impact on development, both in children who grow up to be gay and those who are heterosexuals.

Traditional biases are not easily overcome, as work with lesbian and gay patients has illustrated. Often, coming out does not free them of their own AHB, and in any case coming out is a long process. It can also be a long and challenging process for clinicians to learn about their own AHB. The chapters that follow illustrate how AHB can find its way into the psychotherapeutic setting, the training and supervision of mental health professionals, and the legal system affecting the material and emotional well-being of gay and lesbian patients. For those with severe illnesses, both medical and psychiatric, AHB frequently impedes the delivery of respectful and appropriate health care.

2 AHB IN THE CLINICAL SETTING

This chapter considers a range of therapists' beliefs and feelings, broadly defined as countertransference (Racker, 1968; Levenson, 1983), which can appear and make itself felt during psychotherapy with lesbian and gay patients. Rudolph (1989, 1990) studied attitudes toward homosexuality among counselors. He pointed out that many therapists may not be aware of the unconscious antihomosexual attitudes that could contribute to inconsistent therapeutic positions and actions with their gay patients. He found the evaluative attitudes of counseling professionals toward homosexuality to be divided and contradictory. For example, those surveyed believe in the ability of gay persons to function fully in any situation and yet to be hampered in their performance in certain positions by the very fact of the sexual orientation.

There have also been studies of behavior therapists (Davison and Wilson, 1974) and, more recently, of medical and nonmedical psychoanalysts (Lilling and Friedman, 1995; Friedman and Lilling, 1996). Most of the therapists studied disavowed a pathological model of homosexuality and expressed the belief that being gay is not necessary an obstacle to a happy or a well-adjusted life. In one investigation, however, the same therapists rated homosexual patients negatively on a semantic differential scale (Davison and Wilson, 1974). In another study psychoanalysts were asked to assess case histories identical except for the sexual orientation of the patients. Those analysts showed a tendency to diagnose more frequent and more serious psychological problems when the patient was stated to be homosexual (Lilling and Friedman, 1995). By heightening their awareness of the manifestations of bias in the clinical situation, therapists may be able to monitor themselves and avoid otherwise unfortunate therapeutic mistakes, and achieve a deeper understanding of themselves and their patients.

Freud's (1912) concept of neutrality was based on the notion that the scientist does not judge but merely observes and records facts. In the contemporary literature about psychotherapy, influenced by postmodernism, the idea of neutrality is being replaced by other models that acknowledge the subjectivities of both patient and therapist (Schafer, 1976; Foucault, 1978; Spence, 1982; Levenson, 1983; Butler, 1990: Sedgwick, 1990; Harris, 1991; Lesser, 1993; Schwartz, 1993; Domenici and Lesser, 1995; Magee and Miller, 1995; Drescher, 1996a, b, c, 1998a; Kiersky, 1996). These new approaches ask that therapists learn more about themselves, to become more familiar with their conscious and unconscious attitudes and feelings and the ways in which they may express themselves in therapeutic relationships with patients.

The basic principles of psychotherapy with lesbian, gay, or bisexual patients are those of the psychotherapeutic process in general and are discussed in the vast literature on that topic. While this monograph draws on many aspects of that literature, no attempt is made to review it here. There are also a number of valuable resources on specific aspects of therapy with gay and lesbian patients: Marmor (1980); Stein and Cohen (1986); Friedman (1988); Ross (1988); Isay (1989); Friedman and Downey (1995b); Hancock (1995); Cabaj and Stein (1996); Falco (1996); Magee and Miller (1997); Drescher (1998b). We will first outline some basic themes in AHB, and then draw on some actual experiences and information through clinical vignettes that illustrate commonly occurring problems related to AHB in psychotherapy.

Types of AHB in the Clinical Setting

In 1990, the Committee on Lesbian and Gay Concerns of the American Psychological Association queried a randomly selected sample of members regarding biases in psychotherapy with lesbians and gay men. Responding to the questionnaire were 2,544 psychologists, from whose responses the committee identified 25 commonly occurring themes illustrating bias. Drawing on those findings, as well as other sources, we have identified five patterns of AHB frequently found in psychotherapy:

1. *Pathologizing:* A therapist's belief that homosexuality per se is a form of psychopathology, developmental arrest, or other psychological disorder.

2. *Stereotype, stigma, and misattribution:* A therapist automatically attributes a patient's problems to his sexual orientation without evidence that this assumption is correct; or the therapist focuses on sexual orientation as a therapeutic issue when it may not be essential to the concerns that brought the patient into therapy. A therapist will rely on cultural stereotypes of homosexuality (i.e., gay men are esthetically inclined; lesbians are man haters) as a substitute for knowledge about an individual gay or lesbian patient.

3. *Empathic failure:* Empathy is the process of consciously or unconsciously feeling or understanding, intuitively or intel-

lectually, the internal situation or emotions of another being, who is separate and different from oneself. Empathy implies not only a sympathetic understanding of another who is functioning in a different situation from oneself, but also an ability to see others from their own set of values and points of view. The empathic process has been attributed to projection of one's own psychological presuppositions and functioning. Such projections can, however, lead to a false assumption or conclusion. Empathic failure may be due to a lack of knowledge of countertransference. Whatever its cause, a therapist's failure to recognize a lesbian or gay patient's psychological symptoms and distress can seriously escalate the patient's social stigmatization and antihomosexual self-hatred (internalized homophobia).

4. *Heterosexism:* As defined earlier, this ideological system denies, denigrates, and stigmatizes any nonheterosexual form of behavior, identity, relationship, or community. Heterosexism believes in the inherent superiority of social practices and cultural institutions associated with heterosexuality. This belief system is usually accompanied by a therapist's denial and devaluation of vital aspects of lesbian or gay emotional growth and ignores the development of healthy interpersonal relationships.

5. *Unsolicited attempts to change a patient's sexual orientation:* Without being requested to do so, a therapist may seek to change a patient's sexual orientation by advocating or prescribing heterosexual behavior, or even prohibiting homosexual behavior. The therapist may ascribe relational difficulties to the patient's being gay, rather than to the complexities of a particular relationship.

Each of the five patterns of AHB described can result in lapses from acceptable standards of professional ethics (Brown, 1996). Some lapses are due to simple ignorance of contemporary research data on human sexuality and sexual orientation, lesbian and gay development throughout the life cycle, or the subculture within gay and lesbian communities. Education can address this kind of lack of knowledge, and expert consultation and supervision can help the therapist who is willing to learn about these matters. However, limitations in a therapist's empathy for the experience of lesbian and gay patients frequently result from deeper psychological and psychocultural sources of AHB. Therapeutic empathy is an invaluable instrument, but it is far from infallible. Psychotherapists may be likened to those cultural anthropologists who achieve the goal of exploring unfamiliar ways of life sensitively and cautiously, remaining aware of differences but not assigning value judgments from their own culture to the culture under study. Like such investigators, therapists need to seek to understand how beliefs and practices that may seem strange, anxiety provoking, and even illogical can be coherent, functional, and deeply significant to others. Secure therapists refrain from attempts to impose personal moral values on patients.

AHB in the Clinical Setting: Psychotherapy with Individuals

In this section we present clinical vignettes that illustrate the actual workings of AHB that often occur in clinical practice. The vignettes are composites of case descriptions collected by members of the Committee on Human Sexuality. The composite method was used in order to protect patient confidentiality.

Vignette 1

A 35-year-old homemaker and mother of two consulted a psychoanalytically oriented 45-year-old heterosexual male psychiatrist because of dissatisfaction with her marriage. She had been married for 15 years to someone she felt she never truly loved and with whom she experienced no sense of romantic or sexual vitality. She increasingly found herself erotically attracted to a woman friend. The two women had a sense of deep communication and mutual physical desire. The patient was aware of two sets of problems: she thought that she might be a lesbian, and she found herself considering divorce. She was troubled about the effect that deciding to divorce would have on her husband and especially on her children. She felt it was necessary to explore her feelings in therapy before proceeding. She was assessed by the consulting psychiatrist as suffering from a DSM-IV diagnosis of Adjustment Disorder with Mixed Emotional Features and as having some histrionic personality traits, but not a personality disorder.

In the initial two sessions, the psychiatrist advised his patient not to leave her husband and to desist from "going any further" in her relationship with her woman friend. He explained that he felt that she was acting out unconscious feelings of hostility and conflicted sexuality and that she was tempted to flee impulsively from the "real issues" in her marriage. The patient abruptly terminated treatment. This psychiatrist then sought consultation with a colleague.

Discussion: Evaluating what had happened with his consultant, the therapist realized that his own AHB had influenced him to advocate the preservation of the patient's marriage, had led him to oppose her considering possible other identity choices, and had caused him to disapprove of her sexual attraction to a woman. His treatment recommendation had been based primarily on his personal value system and not on his clinical assessment of the patient. This advice constituted an abandonment of therapeutic neutrality disguised by the use of psychodynamic terminology.

This vignette also illustrates aspects of the therapist's "heterosexism," which can lead to skewed or distorted clinical outcomes and even errors, for example: automatically assuming that a patient is heterosexual and discounting the patient's self-identification as gay or lesbian; devaluing the quality or underestimating the potential worth of a gay or lesbian relationship owing to the privileging of conventional heterosexual forms of relatedness as more desirable; neglecting to take a careful and unbiased sexual history and automatically presuming the patient is heterosexual until he or she states otherwise; and failing to create an atmosphere in which the patient can talk safely about same-sex feelings.

A lesbian or gay patient, sensing a therapist's heterosexist beliefs, may fear the therapist's disapproval. Like the patient just described, many lesbians and gay men leave treatment when they sense such disapproval and do not discuss their reasons for doing so. Some, taking heterosexism for granted both in and outside the therapeutic setting, stay and ignore this aspect of the therapist's beliefs. Remaining in therapy under such conditions generally has deleterious effects on self-esteem. Others may engage the therapist in an effort to change his or her beliefs. Sometimes doing so may be helpful if the therapist is not defensive.

This vignette also illustrates the value to a therapist of requesting appropriate consultation or supervision, ideally before the rupture of the therapy.

Vignette 2

A lesbian patient being treated for depression and her ex-husband, who was not in psychiatric treatment, were embroiled in a custody battle for their five- and seven-year old sons. The woman's therapist, a husband and father from a conservative background, said that the children's interests might be better served if they were placed with her ex-husband. Living with their father, he pointed out, would allow them to have an "appropriate" role model in their custodial parent; they would not have to contend with homophobia from schoolmates and others; and they would be more likely to become heterosexuals. The therapist expressed these views without ever having examined the husband. The patient told her therapist that the children's father had problems with alcohol abuse and had difficulty holding a job because of his poor frustration tolerance. The therapist nonetheless told the patient that it was important for boys to have an "on site" father as a role model regardless of other troublesome aspects of the father's history.

Discussion: The heterosexual father is presumed to be the better parent without exploration of his limitations. This presumption can sometimes result in a therapist's automatically attributing a child's problems to his or her parent(s) being lesbian or gay, without evidence that this is so. This attitude may also reflect the unconscious belief that a gay parent will cause a child to grow up to be gay. A therapist who relies on cultural stereotypes about sexual orientation is likely to oppose child custody for lesbian and gay parents on the grounds that their sexual orientation per se makes them unfit, despite the evidence against this bias (Patterson, 1995; Kirkpatrick, 1996). Even after learning about the significant problems of the children's father, this therapist believed that all other legitimate concerns about the father's fitness to parent were not as important as the mother's homosexual orientation. Because psychiatrists are often consulted by courts in custody battles, this manifestation of AHB often extends beyond the individual therapy situation. Sexual orientation of the parent should not be the chief determinant of the outcome in child custody battles.

Psychotherapy with lesbian patients requires specialized knowledge (Hanley-Hackenbruck, 1993). The therapist was unable to empathize with his patient's desire to raise her children. Further, he was unaware of the literature demonstrating that gay and lesbian parents raise children as well adjusted as those raised by heterosexual parents (Kirkpatrick, Smith, and Roy, 1981; Kirkpatrick, 1987, 1996; Patterson, 1992, 1995; Pattterson and Chan, 1996). He championed the values of the larger society instead of considering those of his parent. In a more general sense, he exhibited problems as a sensitive, responsible therapist.

Vignette 3

A 22-year-old man consulted a psychiatrist because he was preoccupied with many fears. He was preoccupied with and terrified of his "inclination" to engage in homosexual activity. He feared he would "have to" participate in receptive anal intercourse. The psychiatrist diagnosed a mixed personality disorder with schizotypal and obsessional features. The patient's sexual history revealed that he had had exclusively homosexual fantasies since early childhood. His dreams and masturbation fantasies were also exclusively homosexual. He had never actually engaged in sexual intercourse with anyone, male or female. Although he had enjoyed some kissing and caressing with an adolescent male friend, he broke off their friendship because he felt pressured by the man to go further sexually. His concerns about anal intercourse were never explored in therapy.

The psychiatrist, a middle-aged heterosexual man with a fatherly style, advised the patient that a person's sexual identity was usually not fully formed at the age of 22. He suggested that the patient might not be gay at all, particularly because, "unlike most gay men," the patient had not been sexually active at an early age. He then told the patient that avoiding homosexuality might permit the emergence of heterosexual desire. Pointing out that the patient had had no truly intimate relationships, he suggested putting "sexual orientation on hold" and working primarily on the "intimacy problem" in psychotherapy.

Discussion: The therapist's rationale was that abstinence could lead to the emergence of heterosexual fantasy. Most clinicians would disagree. Nor is this supposition borne out by the developmental histories of many lesbians and gay men, a number of whom had practiced abstinence before "coming out." It reflects a once commonly accepted belief that human beings are all heterosexual until proven otherwise (Rado, 1940, 1949; Bieber et al., 1962). Recent scientific studies have invalidated this assumption. Contemporary clinicians now use a paradigm based on diversity of developmental pathways (Bell and Weinberg, 1978; Bell, Weinberg, and Hammersmith, 1981; D'Augelli and Patterson, 1995; Cabaj and Stein, 1996).

There was no clinical evidence to support the idea that the patient should question his sexual interest in men as "inauthentic" because he had not yet been sexually active. There may have been many reasons underlying his decision not to be sexually active, including fear of anal penetration, concerns about infection with HIV, religious beliefs that interdict homosexual behavior, and the conviction that sexual activity should occur only in a committed, intimate relationship. Nevertheless, his sexual fantasy life appears to have crystalized as homosexual. It is worthwhile for a psychiatrist to be sensitive to, and to explore with the patient, the underlying psychodynamic and developmental issues that led to the apparent lack of intimate relationships in his life. In some patients, primitive bodily fears result in terror visualized in the metaphor of anal intercourse or "passivity." There can be many ways to interpret this patient's fears, consistent with his psychosexual organization and structural level (Friedman, 1988). But here the initial interventions were based on stereotyped and stigmatizing bias on the part of the psychiatrist.

This was a complicated, but not uncommon, clinical situation, in which a significant portion of the therapeutic work was devoted to determining the severity of the patient's personality disorder and the extent to which thinking disturbances (such as obsessions) interfered with his functioning. If a patient's personality disorder is severe, then disturbing fantasies and conflicts about sexuality (as well as those regarding other aspects of perceptions of self and others) are to be expected.

If the personality disorder had not been so severe, then the young man's concerns might have reflected fear based on an incorrect stereotype that gay men must have anal intercourse. Similarly, the psychiatrist's formulation seemed to grow out of a preconceived theoretical notion linking gay male sexuality and early sexual activity, rather than from the developmental material presented by the patient. Much more information is needed about the nature of his concerns, which may derive from stereotypes about "typical" gay behavior as well as from other more central psychological issues.

Vignette 4

A gay male social worker had been in psychotherapy with a heterosexual male therapist for a number of years. The patient was in a long-term relationship with a man when he began treatment. Seven years later, when the relationship ended, he described to the therapist how deeply sad and confused he felt about the loss. His therapist commented, "You know, you've always been confused about the difference between a vagina and an anus," failing to address the grief and separation anxiety. The patient became quite anxious and defensive and challenged the therapist to clarify his theoretical position regarding homosexuality. The therapist denied any disparagement of homosexuality in his remark and told the patient that he had misunderstood the therapist's position. The patient decided to give the therapist the benefit of the doubt. A year later, however, when the patient ended a brief new relationship with another man, the therapist raised the issue of how difficult it was to make homosexual relationships work. The patient, remembering the remarks of the previous year, became enraged and felt that the therapist appeared to have an unspoken agenda to change the patient's sexual orientation through disparaging interpretations of homosexuality. Once again the therapist denied the accusation. This time, the patient confronted the therapist with his perception of the therapist's antihomosexual attitude. An impasse ensued that they were not able to resolve. The patient ultimately left treatment because he felt that the therapist was unable to recognize and admit his antihomosexual bias and heterosexist views.

Discussion: Here the patient experienced the therapist's interventions as an unsolicited attempt to change his sexual orientation. The therapist did this indirectly by casting homosexuality in terms of "confusion" and "difficulty maintaining relationships." The question arises, why did this patient remain in psychotherapy for eight years with a therapist who appeared to have AHB? One possibility is that the patient himself had some conscious or unconscious antihomosexual attitudes. When such is the case, as it commonly is because of the patient's own denial or need to please the therapist, the patient's internalized antihomosexual bias may mirror the therapist's overt, although unacknowledged, antihomosexual bias. The unwillingness of the therapist in this vignette to acknowledge his position was an empathic failure that led to the dissolution of the treatment.

Vignette 5

A gay male therapist found himself chronically irritated with a woman patient who described herself as lesbian although she was not sexually active. He challenged her self-identification, wondering aloud what it was based on, since, he felt, "actions speak louder than words." The patient defended her right to claim a lesbian identity, insisting that in her view it was not necessary to be sexually active in order to be a lesbian. She claimed that lesbianism also referred to a certain type of inner experience and perhaps also to a sense of community with other women who shared her personal and political values. She objected to what she felt was an excessive emphasis on sexual activity by males—both gay and straight—in any discussion of sexual identity. She felt that her therapist was guilty of using sexual behavior, rather than subjective feelings, to label one's sexual identity.

Discussion: In this example, the gay male therapist demonstrated a failure of empathy for his lesbian patient. This failure was part of a personal difficulty he had with regard to being empathic with the psychosexual experiences of women and partly due to his lack of knowledge about the development of a lesbian identity. This vignette illustrates an important point: membership in one oppressed group (gay male) does not automatically confer empathy with other disempowered persons (Drescher, 1996c). This patient actively objected to the dismissal of her feelings, experience and knowledge of herself, but fortunately this therapist was able to recognize the countertransferential aspects of his angry reaction. Too often, however, patients are so fearful of their therapists' disapproval or discomfort that they withhold information about their sexuality to avoid confrontations. This kind of avoidance can lead to a vicious cycle in which inadequate disclosure further forecloses the possibility of true empathy, understanding, and acceptance and seriously compromises the effectiveness of the therapeutic work.

Vignette 6

A lesbian therapist, who was herself in the process of struggling with the issue of coming out to family members and colleagues, began treatment of a 19-year-old lesbian patient who had never revealed her sexual orientation to anyone. The patient, diagnosed as having dysthymia and mixed personality disorder with passive–aggressive and obsessional features, had a lengthy history of self-destructive behavior at school and in her personal life. As a result of her repetitive self-defeating character style, the patient had never achieved her academic potential. Furthermore, her love relationships had been fraught with emotional pain and mutual frustration. She longed to be "loved" and understood but, for reasons she could not fully comprehend, consistently undermined all attempts at intimate relationships. She was financially dependent on her parents, who were both described as authoritarian, deeply religious, and highly conventional people who endorsed traditional gender roles and who were intensely opposed to any public expressions of homosexuality.

The therapist encouraged her patient to disclose her sexual orientation to her parents. She did this by communicating to the patient the idea that "honesty was always the best policy." When the patient acted on this recommendation, her parents immediately and violently rejected her. She, feeling destitute and bereft, attempted suicide and was subsequently hospitalized.

After consulting with a colleague, the therapist realized

that she had unwittingly encouraged the patient to behave in a self-defeating and ultimately self-destructive fashion. The therapist's unresolved conflicts about her own homosexuality had influenced her to advocate that her patient disclose her sexual orientation without fully considering the timing and preparing her for the possible consequences of that action for the patient. As a result, the therapist failed to assist the patient in an appropriate manner.

Discussion: This case illustrates two ways in which countertransference issues can lead to empathic failures in psychotherapeutic work with lesbian or gay patients. The therapist's own struggle and uncertainty over coming out affected her advice to the patient about how to proceed with her own coming out. This was a countertransferential enactment. The patient's suicide attempt was also, in part, a concretization of the therapist's own unconscious fear that lesbianism would lead to punishment. Although the lack of acceptance in the patient's home environment was not in itself a contraindication for coming out, the therapist's countertransference caused a serious underestimation of both the young woman's psychopathology and the real consequences of coming out to her family. The vignette also illustrates how narrowly attempting to define the totality of a patient's issues within the paradigm of "coming out" can lead a therapist to ignore the patient's psychopathology as injudiciously as one who overdiagnoses psychopathology in a lesbian and gay patient. In both cases, an overemphasis on sexual orientation can blur the focus on clinical issues of major importance.

AHB in the Clinical Setting: Psychotherapy with Families, Couples, Children, and Adolescents

AHB has worked against clinicians' trying to obtain accurate knowledge of gay and lesbian lives; their identity development; the patterns, styles, and psychological significance of "coming out"; and family life cycle experiences. This lack of knowledge has led to difficulties in providing adequate evaluation and treatment for gay and lesbian adolescents, couples therapy for gay and lesbian couples, and family therapy for both the families of origin and the families established by lesbians and gay men.

Although many of the principles of treatment in these clinical situations are the same as for other patient populations, the impact of AHB on the knowledge, attitudes, and countertransference vulnerabilities of the therapist may limit what he or she can offer to gay and lesbian patients.

In this section, we use clinical illustrations to indicate some of the many ways in which psychiatrists and other psychotherapists can improve their psychotherapeutic effectiveness in these settings by alerting themselves to bias and by acquiring knowledge and skills that will enable more positive interventions.

Vignette 7

An 11-year-old boy was brought for treatment by his parents. His father complained that he and the mother were very uncomfortable with their son's "feminine" behavior. The boy wanted to play the flute, had mostly girls for friends, and was resistant to his father's attempts to involve him in competitive sports. The parents were concerned that the child would grow up to be "homosexual" even though there was nothing to suggest that he had been sexually interested in boys or men. The boy did not meet criteria for gender identity disorder (GID) of childhood in that he had neither a compelling desire to be a girl nor a hatred of his own gender.

The child psychiatry Fellow who was working with the family planned to explore with the parents their gender-role expectations and hopes and fears for their son. Before doing so, she presented the case to her supervisor. After hearing the case, the supervisor suggested that it was not necessary to obtain more family data in order to develop a treatment plan. He commented that the boy would not "make it to heterosexuality" and suggested that the Fellow tactfully prepare the parents for a likely homosexual outcome.

Discussion: Children whose gender-role behavior is not typical in some sense may be pejoratively labeled by their parents. These children may or may not have GID. Sometimes the parents request professional assistance to prevent a child from becoming gay. Here, the child becomes a focus of parental conflicts that may be denied and projected. In situations such as these, assessment of the entire family system is indicated.

Children with GID who require treatment are a discrete and relatively small subset of the larger population of all children who have atypical gender-role interests. Some of the distinctive differences that the clinician must be able to recognize in a GID child include not simply a predominant interest in behavior and activities that are typical of the other sex, but also play interests that are constricted, compulsive, rigid, and not freely androgynous or varied. Children with GID often have intense anxiety as well (Coates, Friedman, and Wolfe, 1991; Zucker and Green, 1993; Zucker and Bradley, 1995). Even among such children, however, it is often not possible to predict future sexual orientation. Although the majority of children with GID become homosexual adults (Green, 1985, 1987), this is by no means always the case (Zucker and Bradley, 1995). Most gay and lesbian adults did not have childhood GID. The patient in this vignette did not have GID. The only way to assess his sexual orientation would have been verbalized sexual fantasies, or reports of sexual behavior, or both. The supervisor's conclusion that the child would not "make it to heterosexuality" reflected his bias and was not supported by data from the clinical situation. Parental chief complaints about the sexual orientation of a child frequently mask conflicts about sexuality and gender role behavior and AHB in one or both parents.

Vignette 8

A 16-year-old male was referred to a psychiatrist because his school grades had precipitously declined over the past five months, despite previous high scholastic aptitude and achievement scores. At the same time, his rebellious defiance of his parents, both professionals, became intolerable to them. He refused to obey parental rules regarding chores, curfew, homework, and religious observances. In response to a sarcastic note left for him by his mother, he wrote back: "Mom, I think I'm gay." Adjustment disorder of adolescence with mixed disturbance of emotions and conduct was diagnosed, and Danny agreed to the recommendation of weekly psychotherapy.

After several sessions dealing with his anger about his parents' "insulting" behavior, the psychiatrist asked the patient if he had any other problems to put on their agenda for therapeutic work. Danny responded, "I think I'm gay, or maybe AC-DC. I absolutely adore Jan—she's 18 and away in college now—and I've loved having sex with her, but now I'm having terrific sex with two of my male friends. What am I?"

The therapist acknowledged the anxiety and confusion that his patient was feeling, but wondered if it was really so urgent that he foreclose "right now" on either exclusive heterosexuality or homosexuality. The patient was startled to learn that some people actually settle on a bisexual life style, while others experience erotic arousal to both sexes at different times but eventually settle into a single-sexual identity orientation. Enormously relieved, he said that he thought he could take his time. He then resumed concentrated therapeutic work on his necessary developmental tasks of adolescence—including, but not limited to, his sexuality.

Discussion: Working with gay and lesbian adolescent sexuality in psychotherapy is much like working with adolescent sexuality in general. The psychiatrist working with adolescents is often perceived by the parents as an extension of their parental authority and values. This is, of course, an inappropriate role for any psychotherapist, particularly when it comes to enforcing parental attitudes and expectations about sexual behavior and orientation. With heterosexual youth, parents often attempt to enlist psychiatric authority to reinforce a variety of attitudes and beliefs, such as sexual abstinence, avoidance of masturbation, beliefs about contraception, pregnancy, and the like. With gay and lesbian youths, parents may attempt to enlist the therapist's authority to reinforce AHB. Thus, to the guidelines for competent therapy with adolescent patients in general one must add the awareness of the impact of AHB on the patient, the family, and the therapist.

While many lesbian and gay adolescents appear to adjust to their same-sex feelings without ever seeking professional help, others are confused about their sexual orientation and may seek psychiatric help to clarify their feelings. Or, as in this case, they may produce a "cry for help" that mobilizes parents to seek help for them. Both diagnosis and treatment may be complex, especially when the family's AHB causes great anguish and tension in the teenager and in the family. It is important for the therapist to understand the development of sexual identity and to help these patients sort out their confusion and distress. Some adolescents are merely experimenting, but others are recognizing erotic feelings and attractions that are predominantly or exclusively homosexual. The therapist should be familiar with the guidelines that have been developed for treating such patients (American Academy of Pediatrics, 1993). Some of these adolescents may be on their way to a bisexual lifestyle.

Same-sex erotic feelings may lead to feelings of shame, self-doubt, fear, and confusion. To make matters worse, while struggling with the internal conflict, some youths feel isolated or cut off both from their peers and from family. Therapists can become a particularly powerful influence to such troubled young persons, who may feel enormous pressure to "get everything settled" and especially not to disappoint parents. It is therefore especially vital for a therapist to be aware of the wide variety of symptoms, defenses, and coping behaviors that an adolescent may adopt. It is important to avoid the pitfall of either overestimating or underestimating the seriousness of the symptoms while missing the desperate need for someone to recognize and help with the task of sorting out the confusion, so that the adolescent can move toward enhanced self-esteem and the integration of a positively valued sexual identity. In this case, individual psychotherapy with the identified adolescent patient was successful. In many cases, it is important for the therapist to recommend family therapy to improve communication and address tensions between the gay or lesbian adolescent and the parents.

Vignette 9

A 17-year-old woman was referred for psychotherapy because of depression, suicidal ideation, and angry outbursts. She revealed to the heterosexual male analyst that she was feeling upset about crushes on other girls. Over the next 10 years she saw the analyst in psychotherapy and analysis and achieved academic and career success. Throughout this time, she presented herself as heterosexual in the community although she had never experienced sexual desire for, romantic fantasies about, or sexual activity with a man. She remained extremely secretive regarding crushes on and sexual attractions to women, telling no one but her analyst. She experienced her homosexual feelings as a problem to be overcome.

The analyst frequently explored possible unconscious motives leading the patient to avoid passionate attachments to men. Neither he nor the patient, however, attempted to analyze the patient's negative attitudes toward being a lesbian. In a subsequent treatment, the patient realized that she had adopted the antihomosexual attitudes of authority figures from her childhood. Associated with this insight was a sense of identity cohesion as a lesbian. She became involved in a love relationship with another women and disclosed her lesbian identity to others.

Discussion: The first therapist responded in a concrete fashion to the patient's stated wish not to be "homosexual" and did not help her to explore her reasons for feeling that way. The negative stereotypes she entertained about homosexuality were reinforced by the therapist because he shared them and did not recognize that they were symptomatic of her internalized homophobia. Analysis of the patient's internalized homophobia in the second treatment led to increasing feelings of self-esteem and security. She became able to use the gay/lesbian subculture as a source of sustenance and support.

Vignette 10

A couple married for 10 years with two girls, ages five and seven, sought therapy because of marital difficulties. The wife, a 35-year-old physician, wished to improve her relationship with her husband, a 40-year-old film maker. He wanted couple's therapy to help him decide whether to stay in the marriage. Both shared many interests and admired each other. Despite deep affection, however, they had not been sexually intimate for four years. The husband explained that this lack of intimacy was because he was gay.

He had been exclusively attracted to males since late childhood but had only a few brief homosexual relationships prior to meeting his wife. In individual therapy at that time the husband's therapist had assured him that he would one day experience heterosexual desire if he met the right person. When the husband was introduced to his future wife by a friend, this therapist encouraged him to pursue the relationship. He discovered that he could engage in sexual activity with her if he imagined she was a man. During the early years of the marriage the couple had sexual intercourse once every month or two. She reassured him that sex was not of great significance and that they were well suited to each other. After the birth of their second child, he began to frequent gay bars and to "cruise," activities he kept secret from her. While attending a discussion group for gay and bisexual men, the husband realized that he was gay. Shortly after, he disclosed this insight to his wife and was surprised to learn that she had long ago realized that this was the case.

A few months before seeking consultation, the husband fell in love with a 25-year-old man. He was now requesting help in deciding whether to remain married or to separate from his wife and come out as gay.

Discussion: This case illustrates how complex issues become in therapy with gay men and lesbians who have denied their orientation for years and started families based on a heterosexual couple model (Buxton, 1994). The husband's earlier, individual therapy reinforced his confusion about his sexuality and his negative beliefs about homosexuality, both of which undermined his self-esteem and led him to deny or suppress important aspects of himself. His therapist had encouraged him to adopt a heterosexual lifestyle. Hence, his gay identity development was delayed until well into his adulthood. At that point, his coming out in the context of a marriage and family had life-changing implications for his wife and children as well as himself.

The transitions can be very painful for both spouses and children. Terminating the marriage may be necessary in some cases for the full psychological and psychosexual development of both partners. If the separation is acrimonious, issues of custody and visitation may become highly charged, with each side trying to enlist the therapist as an ally. Therapeutic neutrality here must be buttressed by lack of bias and possession of accurate knowledge of the literature. For example, a number of studies provide data that warrant the recommendation that the sexual orientation of the parent should not in itself be the basis for psychiatric or legal decisions about parenting (Friedman and Downey, 1994).

Space does not allow for extensive discussion of family therapy here. Issues that are commonly addressed include children's painful feelings due to changes in family structures, communication among family members about sexual and gender role values and expectations, and the need of family members for understanding and support.

Vignette 11

A lesbian couple sought therapy after one of them had an affair with a man. They had been partners for 10 years and, for the last several years, the patient complained about her partner's not meeting her sexual needs. She was as confused by the affair as her partner was hurt by it. She wondered if she was "a closet heterosexual, or maybe bi," but also felt that she would be satisfied if certain changes could be made in their sex life.

The therapist, a 40-year-old heterosexual man, was convinced that the patient was "really" heterosexual. Partly because she was an attractive and conventionally "feminine" blonde who appeared even younger than her chronological age of 35 years, he seriously questioned whether she could really be a lesbian. He encouraged the couple to break up their relationship. Although both had committed themselves to their relationship as a lifetime marriage, they agreed to the therapist's guidance.

After an initial period of grieving and some individual therapy with a woman therapist, the patient found herself again attracted to women. She felt that her affair had been acting out her frustration with her partner's unresponsiveness to her requests to enliven their sexual relationship. She began to date women again, with the goal of making a lifetime commitment.

Discussion: Many psychiatrists have to combat years of conditioning that support the stereotyped belief that gays and lesbians cannot maintain long-term relationships. In fact, many flourishing, long-lasting relationships do exist (Bell and Weinberg, 1978; Blumstein and Schwartz, 1983; McWhirter and Mattison, 1984; Berzon, 1988; De Cecco, 1988; Carl, 1990). Since the couples themselves often have to learn to create their relationship without role models or support, and have to devise their own ground rules and find the reasons to stay together beyond the initial sexual attraction (Cabaj, 1988), they are particularly vulnerable to AHB in the therapist's office when they seek help. In this case, the therapist's AHB and his ignorance of what is currently known about lesbian couples prevented him from performing the essential task of recognizing and validating the strengths of the relationship.

In this example, the psychiatrist took the focus off the relationship and onto sexual orientation. He was not able to identify the affair as acting out, a possibility he almost certainly would have entertained were the couple heterosexual. He may have been uncomfortable with, or lacked skills in dealing with, sexual problems between women. More likely, he was ambivalent about lesbian identity and unfamiliar with the prevalence of bisexual experiences among women. Further complicating matters, he based at least part of his assessment of his patient's sexual orientation on his own response to her as an attractive and "feminine" woman, betraying both his stereotyped image of lesbians and his countertransferential response to his erotic impulses toward her.

AHB in Hospital Settings

All the fundamental issues that we have identified as contributing to manifestations of AHB in the clinical setting can and do also arise in inpatient psychiatric units, where they are complicated by the varying roles and increased number of players. The reactions of the staff, of other patients, and of attending and consultant physicians other than the usual therapist can dramatically affect the treatment of a gay or lesbian patient whose psychiatric crisis has resulted in a hospital admission. The following vignettes illustrate some of the resulting complexities.

Vignette 12

An 18-year-old male immigrant Muslim college student with borderline personality disorder was admitted to a psychiatric facility following a very serious suicide attempt involving a massive drug overdose, hanging, and carbon monoxide inhalation. The patient had recognized his strong homoerotic orientation since early adolescence yet had struggled against its expression because of his deeply held religious views. He had begun having sexual experiences with men beginning at age 17 and had had no sexual activity with females. Marriage was strongly endorsed in this patient's subculture, and his parents applied pressure that he marry. Recently he had proposed marriage to a young woman with the fantasy that marriage would help him become heterosexual. Plagued by ambivalence, he revealed his sexual orientation to her and she rejected him. He then sought and had sexual contact with a man. Feeling intense guilt and profound despair, he made the near-lethal suicide attempt.

Following medical stabilization and transfer to a psychiatric inpatient unit, the patient was assigned to a third-year psychiatry resident. The treatment team sought consultation from a senior attending psychiatrist. The consultant interviewed the patient in the presence of the therapist, other residents, and medical students in a clinical rounds setting. During the interview, this faculty member, an older, married man, questioned whether the patient was truly "homosexual" in light of the fact that he had never participated in sexual activity with females. He advised the patient to abstain from sexual activity with males, and, although not overtly advising him to have sex with females, he endorsed heterosexuality as an appropriate treatment goal. The consultant's rationale for his recommendations was to "provide hope."

The day after the consultation, the patient angrily rebuked the consultant (in absentia) for giving him unhelpful advice. He signed out of the hospital, abruptly terminated psychotherapy, and boarded a plane for his home country. He expressed the belief that he would no longer have sexual feelings and therefore would certainly have no further need of psychiatric help.

Discussion: Many of the issues raised in this case are part of the problems of providing humane and ethical patient care in an inpatient setting, where confidentiality is difficult to balance with the need for the treatment team to share information relevant for treatment, and in teaching hospitals, where students must be exposed to real patients in order to learn. The issues can, however, be intensely painful for gay and lesbian patients, for whom disclosure of their sexual orientation can present serious problems of discrimination, and realistic repercussions for those who were not previously "out." In particular, even the informed consent of a patient such as this one to be interviewed about such obviously personal, sensitive, and deeply conflicted issues in the presence of a group of students and other strangers should probably be regarded as questionable, especially given his seriously distraught state of mind.

In addition, the vignette illustrates some of the issues that are unique to the treatment of lesbian and gay patients. Before choosing to introduce a consultant into this already very tense therapeutic situation, the resident had a responsibility to be informed about the specific expertise of the faculty member. Before accepting the consultation, any psychiatrist has a responsibility to be certain that he or she is an appropriately expert consultant. In this case, the consultant's heterosexism, misinformation, lack of neutrality, and premature "advice" clearly damaged the already precarious therapeutic alliance and probably destroyed any hope that the young man may have felt that therapy could help him.

Sexual values are part of more general value systems that are greatly influenced by cultural and religious factors. This particular patient's sexual value system was affected by the teachings of his religion and by the attitudes regarding sexuality of his family. An opportunity was missed here to help the staff and trainees better understand the contributions of cultural and religious influences to the patient's internalized homophobia. Had more attention been paid to these issues, an appropriate consultation might have been provided and the patient's existential predicament more empathically understood.

Furthermore, an opportunity was missed to help the patient understand the important contributions of AHB produced by cultural and religious influences to his internalized homophobia—as well as to his realistic dilemmas (and probably to educate the staff and students about these crucial developmental factors, as well).

Vignette 13

A 14-year-old boy was admitted to a psychiatric inpatient unit from the emergency room, where he had been treated for a drug overdose. The patient had ingested his mother's benzodiazepine "tranquilizers" with alcohol. Panicking, he told a visiting friend of his mother's what he had done, and was brought to the ER, where his stomach was pumped and he was observed until determined to be medically stable. He was diagnosed as depressed and still at risk for suicide and therefore admitted to the psychiatric unit.

Shortly after admission, he told his assigned psychiatrist, a first-year female resident, that he "had a terrible secret to confess." His secret was that he thought that he was "queer." His history revealed that the patient had experienced exclusively homosexual fantasies since age six. During the past year, masturbation fantasies were also exclusively homosexual. The patient's father and mother had separated when he was six, and his father had an intermittently abusive relationship with the patient and his mother. One week prior to the suicide attempt, his estranged father returned home and had a prolonged screaming argument with the patient's mother. Amidst the invective, the father, an alcoholic, told the mother that her entire family was "no good" and as proof he stated that her only brother was "a faggot." The patient's mother, a Protestant fundamentalist, had earlier told her son about her brother's sexual orientation. Although she did not reject the brother, she considered homosexuality a sin. Before the father was escorted out of the home by the police, he commented that "soon there will be no queers. They will all be dead from AIDS and they all deserve what they get!"

AHB IN THE CLINICAL SETTING

The night prior to the suicide attempt, the patient asked a girl out on a date. She and he had been friends since childhood. He kissed her and felt overwhelmed with guilt and anxiety. He felt that he had "used" his friend, simply to prove to himself that he was not "queer." The next morning, feeling hopeless, he swallowed the pills.

In conference, the entire treatment team sympathized with the boy's distress and formulated the goal of "reassuring him." The staff were instructed to "respond with encouragement to reinforce" any signs of interest in girls that the patient might bring up. The attending psychiatrist, the resident's supervisor, advised him to reassure his patient that adolescence was a time when sexual orientation was uncertain. He might not "really" be homosexual. He should not pay too much attention to his sexual desires—perhaps heterosexual ones would naturally emerge. Shortly after hearing this, the patient attempted to hang himself on the unit. As he was still on suicide precautions, the attempt was forestalled without serious risk to the patient, but a second conference was convened to evaluate the incident.

Discussion: In this vignette, a teenager's suicide attempt was precipitated partly because the clinical staff of an inpatient unit was not sensitive to his cry for help in coping with internalized homophobia. Careful review of the case revealed that the patient was a gay adolescent, living in an antihomosexual environment and afflicted with intense self-hatred because he was gay. Even more immediately damaging, however, was his sense of alienation and isolation. It was extremely difficult for some of the staff to recognize that their "encouragement" only added to this youth's despair. However, a new treatment plan was agreed to in which only staff members who felt able to adopt an accepting and nonjudgmental stance toward the patient's efforts to sort out his troubled feelings about his sexuality were directly assigned to his care. Discharge plans included outpatient individual psychotherapy with the resident who had formed a treatment alliance with him.

The staff requested that there be a follow-up staff conference with the therapist and her supervisor. Ultimately, after extensive outpatient treatment, this patient came to see himself as gay. His depression decreased after he was able to reveal his identity to his mother. Family therapy was initiated, and, even though the father never participated, the patient and his mother were able to work out many important issues. In time, their improved relationship led to the involvement of the uncle in the family therapy; not only did the mother become more accepting of and closer to her brother, but the boy was then able to form a helpful relationship with this positive role model. The psychiatric staff, including the resident's supervisor, who had previously been relatively uninformed about gay and lesbian psychology, learned much from this experience and made concerted efforts to become more knowledgeable. They subsequently included presentations by an invited psychiatrist with genuine expertise in treating gay and lesbian patients, and staff conferences focused on the articles and videotapes recommended by the consultant.

Vignette 14

An experienced male nurse on an inpatient psychiatric unit became perplexed when a psychotic male patient expressed sexual interest in him. The nurse felt that if he were "too nice" to the patient, his kindness might be taken as sexual interest. Moreover, he believed that "homosexuals" tended to be hypersexual and that he might be sexually assaulted.

The psychiatric consultant to the unit encouraged open discussion of the case at a staff meeting. Many of the staff shared stereotypic beliefs, including the fear that lesbians and gay men were promiscuous and likely to react with anxiety and anger when their sexual advances were rebuffed. Psychoeducation proved effective in this situation, and the staff was subsequently able to deal with psychotic gay patients more appropriately and with much less anxiety.

Discussion: Generally, when a patient expresses heterosexual interest in a staff member, there are guidelines readily available to enable staff to deal with these situations as they occur. Discussion of homosexual issues may not occur routinely on an inpatient unit in the way that heterosexual acting out or other topics may be addressed.

When guidelines for dealing with same-sex feelings and enactments are unavailable on inpatient units, staff may resort to stereotypes in their attempts to address the clinical situation. By including discussions of homosexuality with other issues of gender and sexuality in inservice training, unit structures can be maintained and stereotypes dismantled. Such inservice education will result in both better patient treatment and forestall the potential for acting out.

Conclusion

Although AHB is diminishing in the United States, significant problems still exist. One common theme across many disparate clinical situations in which AHB is manifested is denial. Perhaps even more pervasive than denial of AHB is denial of heterosexism.

In this chapter, we elected to focus on gay and lesbian patients more than on bisexual patients for practical reasons because the topic of bisexuality is particularly complex and warrants a separate monograph. The same qualification applies to atypical gender-role behavior and its varied relationships to homosexual orientation. Another area that we realize is important but that we are not extensively discussing is the relationship between religious values and homosexual orientation. Similarly, although many patients that we discuss had primary psychopathology, our emphasis is on AHB in their treatment and not on the diverse psychiatric disorders themselves.

To the degree that we ourselves are aware of bias, we acknowledge a positive attitude toward gay and lesbian patients.

In these turbulent times it is important to distinguish between sound clinical judgment, empathy for people ill used by society, and political advocacy for gay and lesbian issues. Value conflicts between gay and lesbian patients and others in American society are legion and complicate our clinical work. Thus, it may often be difficult for therapists to maintain the empathy toward patients and their significant others that is necessary for optimal psychotherapeutic treatment.

We hope that critical analysis and review of the manifestations of AHB in clinical practice will help practitioners in this difficult task.

3 THE IMPACT OF AHB ON SUPERVISION AND PROFESSIONAL TRAINING

Most students learn psychotherapeutic technique primarily from supervisors who function as their tutors. The role of the supervisor is therefore uniquely important in the education of psychotherapists. Supervision is an interpersonal, interactive relationship in which a trainee forms part of her or his professional identity by a process of identification with the supervisor. Psychotherapists in training often idealize and identify with supervisors in ways that escape immediate notice by either. For example, even experienced psychotherapists may find themselves making comments, expressing emotions or nonverbal behaviors, or even dressing like a valued supervisor who had been a formative influence during training. Just as the parallel process of psychotherapy involves both realistic and idealized conscious and unconscious identifications that the patient makes with the therapist, so too the supervisee will take in much of what the supervisor conveys, for example, implicit attitudes and values along with explicit theories and technical recommendations.

Despite the importance psychiatry places on supervision as a learning tool, and as an essential check on the dangers of losing one's way in the complexities of confusion and countertransference, the processes of supervision and of becoming a supervisor have not been sufficiently studied. What factors make a supervisor helpful and what factors might make him or her unhelpful or even harmful? Just as therapists struggle to overcome difficulties in understanding and helping lesbian or gay patients, so too supervisors struggle to identify inexperience, ignorance, and prejudice. As is true of other types of patients, it is helpful for supervisors to have had some clinical experience working with gay and lesbian patients. Supervisors who lack this experience might profit from consultation with experienced colleagues. Supervisors need to educate themselves about current information and research on the lives, psychological development, sexuality, and identity formation of lesbian, gay, and bisexual people. An explosion has taken place in the area of knowledge about sexual orientation; and supervisors must be aware not only of psychotherapeutic process but also of newly emergent observations about the biological, psychological, and social aspects of sexual orientation. Current empirical findings on sex roles, sexual development, gender identity and role, and sex differences in behavior are also salient.

"Neutrality" is a valid ideal, emphasizing the responsibility we bear as therapists to respect our patients' values that may differ from our own. We cannot, however, leave all our own beliefs and values outside the consulting room (Schafer, 1976; Spence, 1982; Levenson, 1983; Merlino, 1997). Supervisors should discuss the topic of values candidly without attempting to impose their own values. Effective supervision allows supervisees to struggle with their own values and to see how such value judgments can constrict exploration of a patient's issues. Such supervision allows for the therapeutic goals to be spelled out in a frank and collegial inquiry.

The Special Problem of Institutional AHB and Disclosure of Gay or Lesbian Identity ("Coming Out")

Pervasive AHB within institutions affects the attitudes of trainees, supervisors, and consultants toward lesbian and gay patients and colleagues. Even when the official policy of an institution prohibits discrimination, the climate may still discourage intellectually rigorous discourse about the special clinical issues of gay men and lesbians.

Even if AHB is not openly expressed, it may be pervasive. The fact that many gay and lesbian supervisors find it necessary to be in the closet makes it difficult to locate supervisors and role models for gay trainees. While we do not believe that it is necessary for psychotherapy supervisors to be gay or lesbian in order to supervise gay and lesbian trainees, it is helpful and morale enhancing if at least some faculty are openly gay or lesbian.

AHB is still common, and some gay and lesbian people may have sound reasons for remaining in the closet. For example, a lesbian or gay trainee may avoid "coming out" to a supervisor for fear that the supervisor's reaction could adversely affect his or her evaluation, with repercussions in the training program or even in future career opportunities. A heterosexual trainee who is open to examining her or his biases and countertransference reactions may suppress this interest if the supervisor's response is disapproving. A trainee may be reluctant to confront the unrecognized bias of a supervisor who is well intentioned and who may genuinely feel free of prejudice.

A gay or lesbian supervisor might have conflicts similar to those of the supervisee, as might the patient, the third person in the relationship. Unfortunately, countertherapeutic clinical situations may result if the complex psychological processes involved in self-disclosure of sexual orientation are not recognized. One particularly important area that requires careful attention in all clinical situations that involve coming out, is that of confidentiality. Patients have a right to confidentiality and are entitled to expect it from therapists, but the issue of confidentiality in the supervisory relationship is less clear. A guideline for supervisors in the sensitive areas pertaining to sexual orientation is that their supervisory policies about confidentiality be openly discussed with supervisees early in the supervisory relationship.

Vignette 15

A third-year medical student attempted to organize a conference on the biological aspects of homosexuality at his medical school. In keeping with the medical school's policies that student-organized conferences be conducted under the auspices of a clinical department, he sought sponsorship from his school's department of psychiatry. Although the sponsorship was initially given, it was subsequently announced that the student had "misunderstood" the department's position and that sponsorship had never been offered. The student had already arranged for the conference speakers. He subsequently learned that objections to the conference had been raised by highly placed faculty members who took the position that homosexuality was a form of psychopathology. The conference was to feature biological researchers whose data were being presented as refutations of pathological models of homosexuality. Although this medical school had many lesbian and gay faculty members, few were willing to challenge their colleagues in a public forum. The student, however, obtained sponsorship from another clinical department, and the conference went ahead as scheduled.

Discussion: In this vignette, AHB of psychiatric administrative staff would have blocked a conference designed to educate the psychiatric community about homosexuality. The attitude that homosexuality is pathological (see chapter 2, Types of AHB in the Clinical Setting, Theme #1, Pathologizing) was promoted by administrative attempts to forestall an open scientific discussion in which the validity of scientific positions could be aired and discussed.

That a medical student chose to pursue this issue may demonstrate generational differences among gay and lesbian professionals. AHB may influence older gay faculty not to come out to peers or to risk alienating senior administrative staff by supporting gay-related issues. Even faculty known to be gay may feel at risk of being stigmatized if they overtly support efforts to discuss homosexuality in nonpathological models (Theme #2, Stigma).

"Power Differential" Between Supervisor and Trainee

The boundaries of the supervisor–supervisee relationship are often unclear, particularly regarding the question of confidentiality versus reporting and grading of the trainee.

Vignette 16

A fourth-year resident in supervision with a senior analyst presented a new patient recently referred to her. This was the case of a gay man who was also a first-year medical student. The supervisor expressed consternation about this. She told the resident that she did not understand why the student had even been accepted into the medical school. She explained to the resident that homosexuality represented an inability to control one's perverse impulses and that these students had great difficulty controlling their impulses when they entered their third year of training and would be performing physical examinations on patients. The resident, who was not gay, countered that she had worked with gay medical students, residents, and attendings and saw no evidence of the supervisor's views. She felt so uncomfortable with the supervisor's AHB that she requested, and was granted, a change in supervisors.

Discussion: Power differentials, part of the hierarchical structure of most medical settings, can have a strong impact on how AHB is experienced. The one in power, in this case the senior analytic supervisor, may not feel the need to question her own attitudes and beliefs about homosexuality. In this vignette, pathologizing homosexuality (Theme #1) and stereotyping (Theme #2) the gay medical student/patient as one who would not be able to control his impulses are both conveyed clearly. In this case, the resident was able to voice her concerns to her superiors, who used their authority to change supervisors. Unfortunately, not all supervisees are willing to challenge a supervisor's authority. It is not known whether or not the residency training director took the opportunity to confront the analytic supervisor about her attitudes.

If a psychiatric program is to educate trainees to work with gay and lesbian patients, it is important that it provide supervisors who understand gay and lesbian issues. Gay and heterosexual residents and medical students will not feel comfortable opening up about or asking about gay and lesbian issues unless a safe space for discussion is provided.

Antihomosexual Bias in Training Settings

This section of the report addresses manifestations of AHB in various phases of medical, psychiatric, and psychoanalytic training and its potential impact on the intellectual, professional, and social development of trainees. In the process of learning any complex subject, a trainee's level of knowledge, attitudes, and clinical skill will reflect the relative strengths and weaknesses of the curriculum that he or she has been exposed to during medical school and residency. Relationships with mentors, role models, and supervisors, as well as influential articles and books, shape the evolving perspective of students of psychiatry. The attitudes transmitted about homosexuality by teachers may exert a profound influence throughout their students' careers.

With rare exceptions (Cabaj and Stein, 1996, pp. 619–655), there are sparse systematic data describing how the subject of homosexuality is taught in either psychiatric residency or undergraduate medical education programs. Nonetheless, AHB is commonly communicated either consciously or outside awareness in teaching about homosexuality (Drescher, 1995). The examples of AHB cited in this section reflect the combined experiences of the authors, their patients, their supervisees, and their colleagues.

Some incidents of prejudice mirror stereotypes held by the larger culture that are perpetuated by medical teachers under the guise of clinical expertise. Stigmatizing portrayals of lesbians and gay men are frequently presented by psychiatric educators within the metaphors of illness or pathology. Common examples are the comparison of homosexuality to a deficit such as blindness and the claim that homosexuality is always associated with psychopathology. Another is the social prejudice, often presented as a scientific or clinical fact drawn from what is known about normal development, that vulnerable children and adolescents should be protected from exposure to lesbian and gay teachers and counselors.

Regrettably, psychiatric and medical educators often fail to exert decisive, knowledgeable, and moral leadership in this area by openly challenging AHB. For example, a psychiatric teacher and role model implicitly sanctioned AHB by silently tolerating "harmless" antigay jokes. Similarly, in another instance, an attending psychiatrist did not respond at all to a medical student who proclaimed in a teaching group that "gays have no one to blame but themselves for getting AIDS." Members of the professional community who are themselves closeted gay or lesbian faculty or residents are often reluctant to speak out openly for fear of being tainted with stigma, retaliation, loss of professional prestige, or loss of employment and patient referrals.

Constant exposure to overt expressions of AHB in training settings has a profound impact on gay and lesbian medical students, residents, fellows, and faculty members. As might be expected, these people may experience some of the psychological effects of discrimination. These include a sense of isolation, lowered self-esteem, and difficulty integrating professional and personal identities. Many gay and lesbian students, house staff, and faculty remain closeted because they fear that disclosing their sexual orientation will adversely affect opportunities for individual and professional growth.

AHB in Medical School

In a survey of 126 US medical schools in 1992, which had a 65% response rate, Wallick, Cambre, and Townsend (1992) found that the topic of homosexuality received little clinical attention and was inadequately integrated into the main curriculum. On average, only 3.5 hours were devoted to teaching about the topic of homosexuality throughout four years of medical school. Homosexuality was discussed primarily during lectures on human sexuality and, in some instances, only in the context of a discussion of HIV-related illness. Thus, in the latter situation, many medical students learned to associate the concept of a gay identity with a stigmatized and fatal illness.

Townsend, Wallick, and Cambre (1993) assessed support services for gay and lesbian students in 68 American medical schools. With 61 of the 68 medical schools responding, they found that gay and lesbian student groups were more frequently found in the private (67%) than in the public (50%) universities. A significant percentage (40%) of gay and lesbian respondents indicated that they were fearful of being openly gay in their medical schools and that there were no faculty members available with whom they could discuss gay-related issues. Faculty members with whom a student could discuss gay and lesbian issues were more available in the Northeast and West as compared with other regions of the country.

AHB is not always expressed overtly. For example, an absence of any discussion of homosexuality in the medical school curriculum can have the effect of ignoring the particular needs of lesbians and gay men who appear for treatment as patients. Omission sends the message that lesbian and gay men do not exist as patient populations and do not have important medical problems and needs within a particular sociocultural framework.

Restriction of discussions about homosexuality to a framework of illness is also problematic. Students who have no frame of reference for treating lesbian and gay patients other than as examples of psychopathology or as patients at high risk for contracting and spreading AIDS are likely to treat their patients in stigmatizing and prejudicial ways.

Vignette 17

A lesbian third-year medical student tried to organize a lesbian and gay faculty–student organization at her university. She prepared a flyer to be distributed to all the medical students and faculty, and brought it to the mailroom. She asked for a copy of the school's internal mailing list and showed the flyer to the mailroom staff. She was told by a member of the mailroom staff that it was against hospital policy to circulate the flyer because it contained "inappropriate" material (about gay and lesbian matters). The disheartened student discussed the issue with her mentor, a closeted gay male psychiatrist. He was sympathetic to her plight but refrained from making any practical suggestions about what she might do. She went, on her own initiative, to the university's affirmative action office, where the heterosexual woman administrator immediately informed the mailroom staff they were violating the hospital's affirmative action policies by discriminating against lesbian and gay people. The flyer was then mailed without incident, and the lesbian and gay student–faculty group was established.

Discussion: This vignette illustrates several difficulties encountered by lesbian and gay medical students. One is the absence of support groups within the training setting. This student's attempts to organize a support group were met with resistance from a number of quarters. First, the mailroom staff was arbitrarily uncooperative. In this expression of AHB, "usual" rules and operating procedures are invoked to rationalize the suppression of open expression of homosexuality or lesbian and gay issues. Although opposition to the student's efforts came in this instance from a nonmedical source, opposition may come from any level of the administrative or medical hierarchies.

Her second difficulty arose as result of a special problem involving conflicts within the mentor. As it happened, the mentor was himself secretly gay. When she turned to him for support, he responded in an uncharacteristically passive fashion to her plea for help against the mailroom's arbitrary and discriminatory policy. Generational differences in the coming-out process often result in an absence of strong or assertive role models who are needed by lesbian and gay medical students. Although sympathetic to her difficulties, the mentor was unwilling to bring attention to himself by challenging the mailroom's refusal to distribute the flyer. The heterosexual administrator was not similarly constrained. After the formation of the lesbian and gay support group, the student eventually learned from another faculty member that her mentor was gay. The mentor never joined the support group. The student retrospectively interpreted her mentor's actions as a response to his fear of bringing attention to himself as a gay professional.

Vignette 18

A prominent medical school taught its students about homosexuality as part of a course on normal psychosexual development. In one of the lectures, three physicians, a lesbian and two gay men, were invited to talk about treating lesbian woman and gay patients as well as the issues of developing a gay or lesbian professional identity. The physicians responded to a range of questions from the students including how to deal with the health concerns of lesbian and gay patients or how to interact with lesbian and gay people in their personal and professional lives.

One student asked, "Why do I have to know if a patient is gay?" When one of the teachers responded that it was hard to imagine why a physician would be averse to any knowledge about a patient, the student insisted that he did not see the need to talk about it. It was clear from the groans of his classmates that many of them disagreed with him. The gay physician gave an example from his clinical practice of a patient he had treated for recurrent urethritis. Prior to seeing the physician, the patient had been treated by several other physicians for this ongoing problem. However, none of the other physicians had ever suggested treating the patient's lover of many years even though they knew the patient was gay. The standard practice of treating the sexual partner of a patient with an STD was ignored, possibly because the physicians were uncomfortable thinking or asking about the sexual acts (anal intercourse) contributing to the urethritis of their patient.

Discussion: This vignette illustrates several issues relevant to teaching about homosexuality in medical school settings. First, the use of openly lesbian and gay faculty has often been an effective way to diminish irrational anxiety. Lesbians and gay men stop being a mysterious "other" and become members of the professional community, with something to offer to developing physicians. In addition to providing positive role models for lesbian and gay medical students, these physicians can offer a nonthreatening way for heterosexual medical students to approach lesbian and gay medical colleagues and to express their curiosity about the health-care needs of lesbian and gay patients, without fear of bringing stigma on themselves.

Students who feel threatened by nonjudgmental or accepting discussions of homosexuality offer a particular challenge to educators. These students may have strong personal and religious views regarding homosexuality or may simply feel anxious about the subject. It is important that these students not be stigmatized for their views.

It is vitally important, however, to stress in physician education the importance of respectful attitudes and tolerance if physicians are to provide adequate care for minorities, diverse social classes, and various ethnic groups. This position is consistent with the doctrine "First, do no harm." In this vignette, the instructors tried to explain to the student that it was the role of physicians to know as much about their patients as possible. The student's desire not to know that a patient was gay was both accepted and understood by the gay physician but was explained to be inconsistent with the principles of the highest quality of medical care.

AHB in Residency Training

In a survey of training directors by the American Association of Directors of Psychiatric Residency Training (AADPRT) published in 1978, 23% reported that homosexuality was always taught as "pathological" in their programs, and only 5% said that their programs viewed homosexuality as a normal variant of human sexuality. Although almost a quarter of residency training directors felt that homosexuality is always pathological, no training director said that homosexuality would constitute a basis for rejection from the training program. Crowder, in an unpublished survey of residency training directors in 1988, found that 68% of respondents ($N = 100$) felt that homosexuality was not a mental disorder, but 17% viewed homosexuality as a personality disorder.

In a survey of gay and lesbian psychiatric residents ($N = 80$), Townsend et al. (1993) found that 29% of residents from 44 different programs reported that there was no coverage at all of the topic of homosexuality in their programs. Twenty-one per cent of respondents said that their residency programs viewed homosexuality as pathological (in agreement with Crowder's survey of training directors), and 41% said their programs regarded homosexuality as a normal variant of human sexuality.

The APA Committee on Gay, Lesbian and Bisexual Issues (Stein, 1994) has developed a model curriculum for psychiatry residents to learn about homosexuality. In addition to the acquisition of a certain knowledge base, the curriculum stressed that:

> Residents must receive supervision from qualified faculty who are knowledgeable and experienced in working with gay men and lesbians and who represent positive attitudes and clinical approaches to these persons. The importance of visible, qualified, and respected openly gay and lesbian faculty members as teachers and clinical supervisors cannot be emphasized enough. Similarly, supervision should provide the opportunity for gay and lesbian residents to discuss their personal reactions during their training based on their own sexual orientation without fear of wider disclosure or of disapproval. The sexual orientation of the supervisor for these residents is not a major issue as long as the approach to the resident is sensitive and respectful [p. 9].

An important educational matter at major teaching hospitals today is the influence on younger gay and lesbian residents, fellows, and junior faculty exerted by senior faculty and supervisors who are closeted. Prominent educators who are gay or lesbian themselves often fear that disclosure of their sexual orientation will adversely affect their professional standing. Although their reasoning may be sound, and even adaptive if there is overt prejudice in their departments, the necessity of remaining in the closet is demoralizing both to themselves and to their students. It is particularly difficult to obtain accurate data regarding the extent of this phenomenon because closeted professionals fear any form of disclosure. Following are some representative examples of AHB operating at the residency trainee level.

Vignette 19

A fourth-year medical student was interviewed for admission to a psychiatric residency program. After what seemed to be a reasonable, professional interview, his interviewer said, "I'm going to ask you three questions that I ask everybody. First, are you psychotic?" The student said no. "Are you a substance abuser?" No, again. "Are you a homosexual?" The student replied that he was. The interviewer said, "I'm sorry, but I don't think homosexuals should be allowed to become psychiatrists." The student was dismayed.

Discussion: Applicants for psychiatric residency training have reported AHB in the screening interview. One applicant, applying as an openly lesbian woman, was told that a prominent program "had never ranked an openly gay applicant in the past." Another medical student's application included a record of his extracurricular activities in an AIDS clinic and his high-profile involvement in the lesbian and gay medical student group at his university. His interviewer, upon reading this said, "You seem to be a johnny one-note." Ironically, the interviewer was himself known to be gay but not willing to be open about it and certainly not one to join a lesbian and gay professional organization. Interactions like the one just described point to the difficulties faced by openly gay and lesbian students and residents when they encounter older colleagues who are uncomfortable with the students' degree of "outness." Unfortunately, AHB is also demonstrated at times by lesbians and gays in their own professional settings.

In the vignette, the interviewer's rationalization for excluding gay people from training was the association of homosexuality with severe psychopathology such as psychosis and substance abuse. Although this incident took place many years after the removal of homosexuality from the *Diagnostic and Statistical Manual*, the unfounded association of same-sex attraction with illness persists. Although discriminating on the basis of sexual orientation may be illegal in some places, where no such laws exist, antigay discrimination still thrives.

SUPERVISION AND TRAINING

Vignette 20

A third-year, gay male psychiatry resident was attending a seminar on narcissistic and borderline psychopathology taught by a respected senior psychoanalyst. Although the resident was not closeted within the program, his sexual orientation was not known to this instructor, a faculty member on the voluntary staff. The lecturer explained that "all homosexuals had narcissistic pathology" and that she had "never seen a gay patient who did not have a narcissistic personality disorder." The resident felt offended and challenged her view. He pointed out to her that the gay people she treated and on whom she based her opinion were patients who, by definition, were troubled persons seeking help for various problems. Citing the work of Hooker (1957), he suggested that she was seeing a skewed population sample and that her patients were not necessarily representative of the general population of gay men. The teacher stood firm in her opinion until the resident disclosed his own sexual orientation to her. She then became openly embarrassed and commented, "Present company excepted."

Discussion: This vignette illustrates several difficulties encountered by lesbian and gay residents and trainees. The resident had access to data that the instructor did not know or that she chose to ignore. Hooker's research indicated that sexual orientation cannot be accurately predicted from blind assessment of Rorschach protocols. The dogmatic assertion by the instructor of her opinions as facts meant that the residents might have no exposure to the voluminous scientific and research literature that disagrees with her position and on which the 1973 decision to remove homosexuality from the *Diagnostic and Statistical Manual* was based. Similarly, an instructor who believed that homosexuality is not an illness or one who believed that it is a purely biological phenomenon, would be remiss in not explaining to trainees the historical perspectives and trends that had led to the emergence of that position and the alternative theories against which they argue.

Another common experience in training settings illustrated by this vignette is the heterosexist assumption of the instructor that everyone in the room was a heterosexual unless stated otherwise. In that context, the "homosexual" was presumed to be an outsider who could be described in psychopathological terms with impunity. Only when the gay resident spoke up directly did she publicly, at least, modify her position to the residents at the seminar. The resident who speaks up is the exception rather than the rule. Most lesbian and gay residents have been unwilling to challenge the authority of supervisors and teachers who express views like those of that instructor.

The teacher in this setting believed that homosexuality is always pathological. Although her belief is not currently endorsed by mainstream therapists and mental health organizations, it is still held by a significant minority. For that reason, before beginning treatment, it is sound practice for gay and lesbian patients to clarify the therapist's views about homosexuality and psychopathology.

Vignette 21

A fourth-year female resident was treating a 42-year-old married East Indian male who had developed an adjustment disorder with depressed mood in the context of coming out as a gay man and separating from his wife of 10 years. The resident's supervisor was a senior gay male psychoanalyst who was closeted about his gay identity although he was widely assumed to be gay by residents and faculty.

The patient's acknowledgment of his homosexuality was of great psychological and social significance, given his religious and cultural background, yet the supervisor did not encourage exploration of the issue of the patient's coming out. The resident, who was openly lesbian to close friends and peers but not to her faculty, felt anxious and had difficulty concentrating during supervision.

Discussion: This vignette illustrates both the paucity and the importance of appropriate role models for the development of a professional identity among gay and lesbian trainees. The supervisor of this case, who was not publicly open about his homosexuality, reinforced in his resident the sense that one's gay identity is shameful and something to be hidden. As the case progressed, it became increasingly clear that coming out was an adaptive component of the patient's psychological growth. The case also presented an opportunity to explore in supervision how being closeted can compromise the emergence of personal identity. The resident therapist, however, realized that the psychodynamic issues associated with coming out could not be discussed in supervision because of the supervisor's personal difficulties in this area. The fact that she was not completely out as a lesbian herself made the inability to consult the supervisor more burdensome because at this point in her life his discomfort exacerbated hers.

Vignette 22

A senior resident in psychiatry who was out as a gay man was referred a heterosexual 22-year-old construction worker and body builder who had experienced an episode of anxiety. In the second session, the patient expressed concern that the physician seemed to be somewhat effeminate and asked if he was gay. When the physician acknowledged that he was, the patient expressed doubt that a "fag" could help him with his problems. He did not keep his next two appointments and dropped out of treatment. After the patient suffered a second episode of anxiety, he returned to the clinic, where he was treated by another clinician. Eventually, he revealed an episode of prolonged incest with a brother during his teenage years. It was after that period that the patient had become involved with body building. The resident who originally treated the patient recognized that the patient had responded to the disclosure of the physician's sexual orientation with fear of the resurgence of disowned impulses and memories.

Discussion: Here is an example of AHB in a patient, a situation that is extremely challenging for gay and lesbian physicians who are confronted with attitudes of the "oppressor" in the very people they are trying to empathize with and treat. The physician disclosed his sexual orientation without exploring or considering the significance of this intervention to the patient. With more training and introspection, he was increasingly able to relate discussion of aspects of his own life to concerns of the patient and was able, to a greater degree, to treat patients from diverse backgrounds.

Vignette 23

A psychiatric resident, who was out as a lesbian and had passionate feminist sympathies, was referred a bisexual female patient who had fallen in love with a man. The patient had become depressed while trying to work out with her boyfriend the conditions for their marriage since she wanted to have children and he already had children from a previous relationship.

The resident found herself feeling intensely identified with the patient and angry with the patient's lover. She then began to talk to her patient about her belief that bisexuality is not a natural state but usually represents incompletely acknowledged homosexuality.

Her supervisor, an experienced male therapist, knowledgeable and comfortable about issues of sexuality and gender, pointed out that the resident appeared to have lost the appropriate distance necessary to maintain an effective therapeutic relationship. With her supervisor's support, the resident was able to assume a more therapeutic stance with the patient.

Discussion: This case illustrates a common situation in psychotherapy when a young, idealistic trainee with sympathy for a patient loses appropriate objectivity. The resident had gone through a phase in her own life during which she had thought of herself as bisexual before fully acknowledging her homosexuality. In retrospect, she had never felt emotionally attracted to men. Although she had found sex with them pleasant, it had never been deeply exciting to her. Her life experiences and interests were almost exclusively lesbian.

Because of her failure to see the patient as possibly different from herself, she did not get enough history from the patient to realize that this young woman genuinely had attractions and excitement with both men and women. This error of omission was compounded by a moralistic stance about the patient's relationship with a man.

Although this particular treatment was able to be turned around with timely supervision, there will be occasions when beliefs firmly held by a therapist in training will not yield to additional information and discussion. In these situations reassignment of the case may be required.

AHB in Psychoanalytic Training Programs

Antihomosexual bias in psychoanalysis has a history that illustrates the interweaving of scientific theories and their political and social consequences. Freud himself did not feel that homosexuality per se should exclude qualified candidates from obtaining psychoanalytic training and wrote as much in a private letter to Ernest Jones (Lewes, 1988). Subsequent generations of analysts, however, disagreed strongly (Rado, 1940; Bieber et al., 1962; Socarides, 1968; Ovesey, 1969; Hatterer, 1970) and characterized homosexuality as a form of psychopathology whose presence in a person was inimical to one's becoming a qualified psychoanalyst because of the presence of early preoedipal narcissistic character difficulties. As a result, many analytic institutes routinely excluded from acceptance for training all openly homosexual applicants (Drescher, 1995; Isay, 1996; Magee and Miller, 1997). Similarly, analysts who came out as gay or lesbian after obtaining training were unable to become training and supervising analysts in these institutes. Thus, the conflation of unproven but widely accepted psychoanalytic theories with heterosexual cultural prejudices led to the exclusion of gay and lesbian physicians and psychotherapists from analytic training for many years after homosexuality was removed as a diagnosis from the DSM.

The theoretical assumption that homosexual people invariably suffer from severe character pathology was contested by a number of psychoanalysts including Lief (1977), Mitchell (1978, 1981), Marmor (1980), Stoller (1985), Morgenthaler (1984), and Friedman (1988). It was Isay (1989, 1991, 1996), however, who challenged the historical exclusion of gay and lesbian persons from the training institutes of the American Psychoanalytic Association (APsaA).

After several years of controversy within that organization, the APsaA passed an official statement in 1991 stating that it "opposes and deplores public or private discrimination" based on a person's sexual orientation and that admission to its training institutes should be based on "careful evaluation of integrity, analyzability, and educability, not on presumptions based on diagnosis, symptoms, or manifest behavior" (American Psychoanalytic Association, 1996). Currently, an APsaA Committee on Issues of Homosexuality exists to monitor and deal with any prejudice against lesbian and gay candidates or members in the organization and its training institutes (Roughton, 1995).

Vignette 24

A gay male second-year candidate in a psychoanalytic institute took a course on theories of child development from a well-respected senior analyst. The instructor expressed the view that sexual orientation was independent of psychopathology; he was known to have defended the admission of gay candidates at the local institute level. Much to the candidate's surprise, normal childhood development was described by the instructor as following a single path of resolution of the Oedipus complex, resulting in an object choice that was heterosexual.

Discussion: Well-intentioned psychotherapists, including faculty at major educational institutions, may hold internally contradictory views involving sexual orientation and sexual identity (Friedman and Lilling, 1996). It is fairly common for clinicians to express liberal attitudes without having reevaluated intellectual assumptions to which they were exposed further back in their educational development. In this case, the candidate spoke to the instructor after class and drew attention to the instructor's failure to consider alternative normal developmental paths. A search for literature clarifying this issue led to the collaboration of the candidate and the instructor on a paper they presented at a local analytic meeting.

Vignette 25

A lesbian candidate engaged in a highly successful analytic treatment with a 35-year-old patient in a committed lesbian relationship was presenting the case in a process course led by a female training analyst. All went well until the candidate presented the patient's desire to become a mother and her evolving plan to undergo artificial insemination by donor in order to have a child with her partner. At this point, the faculty member began to advise interpreting this plan as "acting out." When queried, she explained that for normal development to occur children need two parents, one of each sex.

In this case, the training analyst was not responsive to discussion and respectful confrontation by the candidate. However, because the candidate had the support of the equally senior analyst supervising the case, she was able to disagree openly with the course instructor without penalty. Several years later, the instructor approached the candidate, now a new member of the institute faculty, and told her she had changed her mind about what constitutes an emotionally healthy family.

Discussion: This vignette illustrates an instance of heterosexual cultural bias which has the possibility of doing harm because the person expressing the bias is in a position of authority and is assumed to be well-informed. The training analyst chose to ignore the social phenomenon of millions of women raising children without men living in the household and may not have been aware of studies demonstrating that children being raised by lesbian mothers do not differ in gender identity, early signs of sexual orientation, or behavioral problems from children conceived in conventional marriages and raised by divorced heterosexual women (Kirkpatrick, 1987, 1996).

Conclusion

Available evidence from surveys and anecdotal reports identifies significant problems in the way we currently teach psychotherapy trainees about homosexuality. The topic of homosexuality receives too little attention and is not well integrated into medical school or residency training curricula. Standard psychiatric texts often present an incomplete and biased view of the topic.

We believe the following suggestions would address some of these problems:

1. A modern curriculum that is nonjudgmental should be integrated into a human sexuality course for mental health workers in training and for medical students.

2. Psychological and social aspects of homosexuality should be taught in classes or seminars on human sexuality, and not pathologized, and should be included in the parts of the curriculum wherever relevant.

3. Curricula should create possibilities for trainees to be exposed to the perspectives of the lesbian and gay subculture by providing the possibility of contacts with openly gay teachers and supervisors and through introducing students and residents to the literature on homosexuality within a historical context.

Therapists, like all other people, are influenced by the values of their predominantly heterosexual culture. It is important for mental health professionals to be aware of their own beliefs and feelings about homosexuality, as they can have an influence in clinical practice, with colleagues, and in supervision. Social and personal values have a powerful impact on attitudes and thinking about homosexuality.

4 LEGAL ASPECTS OF ANTIHOMOSEXUAL BIAS AND MENTAL HEALTH

This chapter explores some of the history of the relationship between the law and psychiatry, with an emphasis on the impact of the judicial system on the mental health of lesbian and gay patients. Clinicians working with patients who identify themselves as lesbian or gay are often unaware of the relevant legal issues and their wide-ranging effects, and such lack of knowledge can handicap or distort both empathy and effective therapeutic intervention. Furthermore, the law as it involves sexual orientation has been influenced by mental health professionals (Greenberg, 1988). The legal system has yet to keep pace, however, with the dramatic revisions made by mental health professionals about homosexuality. Psychotherapists are often involved in legal conflicts in which homosexuality may assume a prominent role. For these reasons, we discuss legal issues related to AHB.

Discrimination against homosexuality has been so pervasive in American culture that, even today, antihomosexual bias is seen by some as a sign of civic mindedness. Since the 1970s, however, progress in the area of basic civil rights has advanced, fueled by legal challenges to discrimination against lesbians and gay men. As cultural attitudes change and the definitions of "traditional" norms are transformed, conservative institutions such as the fields of mental health and the law tend to follow suit, albeit slowly.

Prior to the deletion of homosexuality from the *Diagnostic and Statistical Manual* of the American Psychiatric Association (Bayer, 1981), persons engaging in same-gender sexual relations (or who simply identified themselves as "homosexual") were characterized as criminals or deviants by many in both the legal and the psychiatric professions. Prominent psychiatrists, such as Hirschfeld, Freud, and Ferenczi (see Bullough, 1979; Abelove, 1985; Lewes, 1988; Stanton, 1991), had opposed the criminalization of homosexuality earlier in the century, but the first edition of the *DSM* (American Psychiatric Association, 1952) classified homosexuality among the sociopathic personality disorders, a diagnostic categorization that revealed contemporary prejudice against homosexuality in both medical and legal lexicons.

The classifications of homosexuality by American psychiatry and by the law began to diverge at the time of the second edition of *DSM* (American Psychiatric Association, 1968), when the diagnosis of homosexuality was reclassified as a sexual deviation, rather than psychopathy. Since then, the legal and psychiatric approaches to a nonconforming sexual orientation differed on the basis of etiologic assumptions. Whereas mental health clinicians attempted to treat homosexuality as a developmental abnormality requiring therapy, the criminal justice system viewed homosexual behaviors as criminal and aimed at deterrence by incarceration and other punitive measures. At times, psychiatrists and psychologists were involved in decisions within the legal system. For example, on the basis of psychological evaluations, persons classified as "homosexual" were legally discharged from military service or deemed ineligible to immigrate to the United States. Futhermore, the assumed etiology of developmental "deviance" rationalized policies under which persons could be denied employment or residence (McCrary and Guitierrez, 1980). After all, many reasoned, how could one hire known felons or deviants to teach children or to work in the Federal Bureau of Investigation?

Privacy and the Right of Association

Legal prohibitions against sexual conduct perpetuate widespread obstacles to intimacy in same-sex couples. Effective clinical practice with patients who are lesbian or gay requires an understanding of privacy issues and the ramifications of laws that attempt to prohibit or regulate homosexual activity.

Private, consensual, homosexual sexual acts remain a crime under sodomy laws in 24 states—approximately half the United States (Thornton, 1995). While sodomy laws are generally enforced in prosecutions for solicitation, they leave all gay men and lesbians vulnerable to classification as criminals. Sodomy laws are discriminatory, mainly because they are enforced selectively to deter same-sex relations and are rarely, if ever, used against heterosexual couples, to whom in theory they also apply. In 1986, the US Supreme Court reviewed a challenge to Georgia's sodomy law in *Bowers v. Hardwick*. In a five to four decision, the Supreme Court upheld a State's right to prohibit consensual homosexual sodomy, even in the privacy of one's own home.

In upholding Georgia's statute, the Supreme Court admitted its reliance on traditional prejudices against homosexuality as the rationale for continuing legal prohibitions against private homosexual activity between consenting adults. The majority opinion of the Court stated that their decision did "not require a judgment on whether laws against sodomy are wise or desirable" but was based on the "ancient roots" of proscriptions against homosexual consensual sexual activity and a long-standing condemnation of those practices in "Judaeo-Christian" moral and ethical standards (*Bowers v. Hardwick*, 1986). Thus, the Court essentially cited the existence of AHB as a justification for continuing the proscription.

The dissenting opinion in *Bowers v. Hardwick* strongly criticized the underpinnings of the majority's decision, however: "An individual's ability to make constitutionally protected 'decisions concerning sexual relations' . . . is rendered empty indeed if he or she is given no real choice but a life without any physical intimacy" (*Bowers v. Hardwick*, 1986). The dissenting opinion emphasized that, in addition to adhering to an extremely restrictive view of the right to privacy, the majority opinion neglected current evidence from research on homosexuality. Justice Blackmun, citing amicus briefs filed by the American Psychological Association and the American Public Health Association, wrote, "Despite historical views of homosexuality, it is no longer viewed by mental health professionals as a disease or a disorder." He argued further along lines of legal precedent that "[n]o matter how uncomfortable a certain group may make the majority of this Court . . . [m]ere public intolerance or animosity cannot constitutionally justify the deprivation of a person's physical liberty" (*O'Connor v. Donaldson*, 1975). The latter principle has been historically applied in the legal system to cases involving other discriminatory attitudes such as racism. In *Palmore v. Sidoti* (1984), for example, the Supreme Court declared: "The Constitution cannot control such [racial] prejudices but neither can it tolerate them." In that case, a white mother retained custody of her child from her first marriage to a white man after entering into an interracial remarriage, despite the claim that the child might be subjected to a variety of stresses due to racial discrimination. The same principle was applied in *Wisconsin v. Yoder* (1972), where the Supreme Court emphasized that: "[a] way of life that is odd or even erratic but interferes with no rights or interests of others is not to be condemned because it is different." In that case, the Court held that the state's interest in compulsory high school education had to give way to the competing claim of the Amish that schooling after the eighth grade threatened their way of life.

A decade after the *Bowers v. Hardwick* (1986) ruling, the Court's decision in *Romer v. Evans* (1996) indicated a willingness to begin to afford some constitutional protections to gay men and lesbians. This case involved Colorado's "Amendment 2," which precluded all legislative, executive, or judicial action (at any level of state or local government) aimed at protecting persons from discrimination based on sexual orientation, conduct, or relationships. In a six to three decision, the majority held this amendment to be unconstitutional. The majority thought that the sheer breadth of the amendment raised the inevitable implication that it was born out of animosity toward this class of people. The majority held that such status-based classification not only was a denial of equal protection guaranteed under the Fourth Amendment but also lacked any rational relation to a legitimate state interest.

Psychiatrists and other mental health practitioners are often sought out by a variety of patients whose lives are adversely affected by AHB, as reflected in court decisions such as these:

1. In *England v. State of Texas* (1993), a lesbian was denied employment as a police officer because of the state's antisodomy law.
2. In *Appeal of Pima City Juvenile Action* (1986), the sodomy law was used as a rationale for finding a man with a bisexual orientation unfit to adopt children.
3. In *Mississippi Gay Alliance v. Goudelock* (1986), the state's sodomy law was used to support a newspaper's refusal to print advertisements for gay services, counseling, and legal aid.

In such circumstances, psychiatrists must be able to distinguish realistic responses to AHB from such mental conditions as anxiety disorders. Friedman (1988) has noted that irrational antihomosexual attitudes prevalent in contemporary culture often lead to painful emotional burdens for patients, their families, and their therapists. As carriers and enforcers of bias, legal issues are not esoteric matters limited to the legal system, but directly influence the mental health of patients.

Institutions and Employment

"Coming out" as a gay man or lesbian may translate into rejection by family or friends, loss of employment, denial of promotions, or eviction from one's home (Harvard Law Review, 1985). Consequently, federal and state antidiscrimination statutes have expanded over the years to include sexual orientation in the provisions to guarantee protection against discrimination based on race, ethnicity, religion, gender, age, or disability. At this point, however, only nine states (California, Connecticut, Hawaii, Massachusetts, Minnesota, New Jersey, Rhode Island, Vermont, and Wisconsin) and the District of Columbia have laws that outlaw discrimination based on sexual orientation. No federal laws to date prohibit discrimination based on sexual orientation in housing, education, or employment (Achtenberg, 1987).

The United States military is highly influential because it is the largest government employer. Historically, military regulations have required harsh punishment for homosexual behavior. Since World War II, the policy has shifted to systematic discharge and sanctions levied against persons who simply identify themselves as lesbian or gay (Rubenstein, 1991). As in the legal system, the application of these regulations is egregiously unequal. Although the military regularly implements this policy with lesbian, gay, and bisexual personnel, it has rarely prosecuted persons for heterosexual misconduct or sodomy (United States General Accounting Office,

1992). In the mid- to late 1990s, women successfully brought actions charging sexual harassment against male officers, and the resulting national attention may result in some changes in this inequity.

The Department of Defense defends antihomosexual policy on the basis of "the [negative] effect of homosexuality on factors such as discipline, good order and morale" (United States General Accounting Office, 1992). The military's criteria for prosecution of lesbians and gay men, however, do not require evidence of homosexual behavior. Members of the military can be discharged for simply announcing their homosexual orientation, regardless of whether they act on it. Consequently, the barriers to managing same-sex desires may prove formidable for military personnel.

There is no right to privacy between patient and psychiatrist in the military. This means that psychiatrists and other mental health professionals are obliged under military regulation to inform commanding officers of admissions of homosexual feelings that may surface in therapy. This lack of patient–physician confidentiality leaves little recourse for personnel who are struggling with an emerging identity as gay or lesbian. An "outed," celibate, lesbian or gay man can find his or her career in ruins despite a lack of evidence of engaging in homosexual behavior and regardless of a distinguished service record (Rivera, 1991).

The military's policy toward lesbians and gay men closely parallels its discriminatory racial policies levied against African Americans in the Armed Forces prior to 1948 (Rubenstein, 1991). Specifically, it was once believed that desegregation of the military would adversely affect the military's morale (United States General Accounting Office, 1992). In that era, one United States Navy memorandum asserted that the enlistment of "Negroes", other than as mess attendants, would lead to disruptive and undermining conditions (Rubenstein, 1991).

Between 1980 and 1990, approximately 17,000 people with homosexual orientations were discharged by the military

(United States General Accounting Office, 1992). In 1990, the financial expense to replace the discharged persons was estimated by Congress's General Accounting Office to be a minimum of $27 million per year, not including court costs and other expenses (United States General Accounting Office, 1992). The GAO report noted that many persons discharged under this exclusionary policy had exemplary records and held important positions within their units. The mental health costs of this policy have not been reckoned. Military psychiatrists have reviewed the data in the military archives and court cases and have concluded that the evidence does not support the stated motives for excluding gay men and lesbians from military service (Jones and Koshes, 1995). The impact of the Clinton administration's 1993 policy of "Don't ask, don't tell, don't pursue" was to increase the number of these discharges (Shenon, 1999), thereby reinforcing the need for lesbians and gay military personnel to remain secretive. Some of the numerous challenges to the constitutional underpinnings of this regulation have been upheld and others are under consideration.

Vignette 26

A young, gay male psychiatrist entered military service as a doctor and an officer. He was assigned the duty of screening candidates for military service to determine their psychiatric fitness. Unofficially, his job was to detect and weed out gay men and women. Because people rejected for homosexuality suffered severe prejudice, he felt it important to prevent these consequences by finding other legitimate reasons for their rejection. However, when he discovered gay candidates who strongly desired to serve in the military, his self-assigned task was to determine whether they were capable of adapting to the pressures that a closeted gay man would experience in the military. If he believed they could succeed, he approved their papers.

Discussion: This psychiatrist chose to juggle military and clinical ethics. Military policy poses a difficult dilemma for many mental health professionals employed by the Armed

Forces. The APA's ethical guidelines require that "a psychiatrist should not be a party to any type of policy that excludes, segregates, or demeans the dignity of any patient because of ethnic origin, race, sex, creed, age, socioeconomic status, or sexual orientation" (American Psychiatric Association, 1993, p. 3). Psychiatrists and other therapists who work in military settings may find themselves facing the ethical dilemma of being asked to support military policies that discriminate against, and that may adversely affect the mental health and well being of, the service personnel under their care.

Marriage and Spousal Benefits

Marriage is a powerful social institution devised to bolster stability by reinforcing the strength of nuclear family relationships. The myriad privileges afforded to married couples are extensive and may be taken for granted by those able to marry legally. Laws prohibiting people from marrying members of their own sex mean that lesbians and gay men are denied economic, social, and legal privileges available to married heterosexuals in our society (Achtenberg, 1987; Sullivan, 1997). These include health insurance benefits for partners, spousal pensions, and disability or social security benefits for partners. Without official bereavement leave or sick time, caring for an unemployed and ill partner who has no health insurance can often deplete a couple's material and emotional resources. Lesbian and gay couples are not entitled to the income tax deductions or exemptions that are afforded to married couples. Moreover, gay or lesbian partners have no legal right to inherit each other's property without extensive estate planning, and they may not be able to take part in critical decisions regarding medical treatment without properly executed health care proxies. Although legal planning can prevent many difficulties, it cannot achieve rights equal to those of married couples, and the legal agreements that are set up still remain vulnerable to challenges and technical errors. Similarly, while our immigration laws provide that a married spouse who is a citizen or permanent legal resident may file for legal immigration status for a spouse, immigration rights do not apply to a same-sex life partner.

In 1993, the Hawaii Supreme Court held that not allowing same-sex couples the right to marry may violate the equal protection clause of the Hawaiian constitution: this exclusion results in discrimination on the basis of sex (*Baehr v. Lewin*, 1993). On remand, the trial court found that the state had failed to prove that the marriage statute denying a marriage license solely because the applicants were of the same sex (*Baehr v. Miike*, 1996) furthered a compelling state interest. Increasingly, states have responded by passing laws that outlaw same-sex marriages (National Gay and Lesbian Task Force, 1997). The Federal government has also outlawed recognition of same-sex marriages by federal agencies. The government's opposition to helping lesbians and gay men build committed relationships is referred to as "The Defense of Marriage Act" (104 Public Law 199, 110 Stat. 2419, 1996), implying that granting gay men and lesbians equal legal recoginition of their unions would attack and weaken stable, heterosexual married couples.

Clinicians are often called on to deal with the consequences of the present state of legal affairs denying same-sex relationships. Working with lesbian and gay couples requires that therapists know something about the mental health burdens imposed by such legal complications as the need for estate planning, health proxies, tax law, and insurance benefits. Heterosexual therapists who may take the legal privileges of marriage for granted need to understand how their lesbian and gay patients living in long-term, committed relationships must make alternative arrangements.

Custody, Adoption, Procreation, and Visitation

There is a growing recognition in both psychiatry and the legal system of the custody rights of gay and lesbian parents

(Hunter, 1991) as well as of the benefits of adoption of children by same-sex life partners (Bonauto, 1993). Psychiatrists and other mental health professionals have made significant contributions to this growing acceptance of nontraditional family structures (Miller, 1979; Golombok, Spencer, and Rutter, 1983; Bozett, 1987; Green and Bozett, 1991). In fact, studies have shown that the children of lesbians are no different from the children of heterosexual solo parents in terms of peer popularity and adjustments (Kirkpatrick, Smith, and Roy, 1981; Green et al., 1986; Gottman, 1990). Although many court decisions continue to go against homosexual solo parents, a number of courts are deciding that sexual orientation should not restrict a parent's visitation or custody rights.

Major progress was made when several states established that sexual orientation does not of itself imply unfitness of a parent in a contested custody proceeding. In *Bezio v. Patenaude* (1980), a pathbreaking case, the Massachusetts Supreme Court held that sexual orientation per se is not evidence of parental unfitness and that an adverse impact on children must be demonstrated. Similarly, in *Cabalquinto v. Cabalquinto* (1986), the Washington State Supreme Court held that being in a gay relationship was not sufficient grounds to justify limiting a father's visitation rights. Courts are now increasingly being asked to focus on continuity of care and the quality of the relationship between each parent and child when deciding which parent can better meet the needs of the child.

Despite some progress, lesbians and gay men often encounter legal challenges to their requests for custody and visitation rights. All too often, divorced gay or lesbian parents can expect to lose custody of a child solely because of their homosexual orientation, often to the exclusion of the most important factors determining the child's best interests (Falk, 1989). A major factor determining attitudes of judges and clinicians making custody recommendations is a tendency to fall back on societal or personal prejudice, rather than on objective data. While sexual orientation per se may not be the manifest reason for judging a parent unfit, living with a same-sex partner remains a criterion to deny custody based on "the best interests" of the child. The Sharon Bottoms case stands out as a example. In *Bottoms v. Bottoms* (1995), the Virginia Supreme Court reinstated an award of custody of a child to the grandmother over the objection of the mother, who was living with her same-sex partner. The court held that it was appropriate for the trial court to recognize that "the social condemnation attached to such an arrangement will inevitably affect the child's relationships with its peers and with the community at large."

Clinicians treating lesbian and gay parents can be more effective when they are knowledgeable about the relevant issues. Mothers who identify themselves as lesbian are not different from solo heterosexual mothers in child rearing practices, with the exception that lesbian mothers tend to make greater efforts to provide their children with male parental figures (Kirkpatrick et al., 1981). Mothers who are lesbian have been found to be more self-confident, independent, composed, and self-sufficient than their heterosexual counterparts (Thompson, McCandless, and Strickland, 1971) and to demonstrate unusually high levels of motivation compared with other mothers (Moses and Hawkins, 1982). Psychiatric consultants can be especially helpful to the judicial system in dispelling pejorative myths regarding sexual orientation and parental skills and providing available scientific data. They can help courts fashion decisions that are genuinely in the children's best interests by assessing parental abilities in a balanced manner. Psychiatrists should also be prepared to help patients who present with clinical problems in reaction to such profound losses as the denial of custody and visitation rights.

Conclusions

The legal system is confronting a growing number of challenges to discrimination against gay men and lesbians.

Advances in the approach to cases involving lesbians and gay men are being made in diverse areas of the law. Discrimination based on sexual orientation is still condoned, however, and even encouraged, by many social institutions. It is critical that the clinician treating patients who identify themselves as gay or lesbian (or who have homosexual inclinations) be knowledgeable about the many legal issues that may influence their health and well-being. Such knowledge and expertise are mandated by ethics and good clinical practice alike.

5 HIV AND AHB IN MENTAL HEALTH

AHB and Bias Against Persons with AIDS in Society

"AIDS," Sontag (1988) writes, "has turned out, not surprisingly, to be one of the most meaning laden of diseases" (p. 99). These meanings have not been neutral. For the most part, they have been deeply negative, with connotations of immorality, pollution, and punishment regarding those infected. In some instances, however, the description of people with AIDS has aroused empathy and a better understanding both of the disease and of gay and lesbian persons.

In the search for historical antecedents to society's response to HIV, the example of leprosy is particularly illuminating. As one AIDS patient said, "The nurses are scared of me; the doctors wear masks and sometimes gloves. Even the priest doesn't seem too anxious to shake my hand. What the hell is this? I'm not a leper" (Kleinman, 1988, p. 163). Attempting to describe the extent of his own experience of rejection, this AIDS patient invokes the image of the leper, the paradigmatic social outcast. Although leprosy has long been synonymous with stigma, this was not always the case. For example, in the 1840s when leprosy was still encountered only rarely among Hawaiians, lepers were not stigmatized. In the 1850s and 60s, when a surge in leprosy cases coincided with an influx of Chinese immigrants, who competed for local jobs and were viewed as an inferior race, blame was placed on the "inferior but ostensibly threatening minority of Chinese coolies" (Waxler, 1981).

Because AIDS first became known in America as an affliction of gay men, the bias that gay men faced was soon shared by the illness itself. From the disease's entrance into American consciousness as GRID, or Gay Related Immune Deficiency (Shilts, 1987a), the threads of meaning of AIDS and homosexuality have been closely intertwined. Homosexuality and AIDS became, and to some extent remain, coterminous in the American imagination. A semantic equivalence was struck between the illness and those at risk, thus, leading one Houston mayoral candidate to declare "AIDS is spelled G-A-Y" (Shilts, 1987b). Having AIDS thus became something akin to being gay, with all the stigma that designation entailed. Once such a semantic bridge was built between homosexuality and AIDS, the stigmatization could move in either direction, resulting in increased bias against gay men, viewed as likely to have AIDS, and against AIDS patients, viewed as likely to be gay (Herek and Glunt, 1988).

The early spread of AIDS in the United States was, consequently, associated with an intensification of AHB. Sontag (1988) explains, "Epidemics of particularly feared illnesses always provoke an outcry against leniency or tolerance now identified as laxity, weakness, disorder, corruption: unhealthiness" (p. 10). A review of 53 national and international surveys conducted between 1983 and 1988 found that one half of Americans surveyed felt that the epidemic had set off a wave of antihomosexual sentiment and was leading to unfair discrimination against gay people (Blendon and Donelan, 1988). The review's authors continue, "People admit these tendencies in their own behavior. One in 12 nationally and 1 in 8 in the South say they are already making efforts to avoid personal interaction with homosexuals" (p. 1023). A 1986 Gallup poll showed that public support of gay rights legislation had dropped to its lowest level since 1977 (Royse and Birge, 1987). This decreased tolerance may have led to a worsening of violence against gay men and lesbians, indicated by the growing number of reported incidents of antihomosexual assaults and harassment from 4946 in 1986, to 7008 in 1987 (Blendon and Donelan, 1988, p. 1023). Being diagnosed with AIDS carried the danger of being identified as gay, with all the accompanying social stigma. In the general public, stigma for presumed homosexual orientation was added to the terror of the AIDS-related illnesses.

AHB and AIDS Bias in Health Care Professionals

The adverse effects of stigma on both the government's management of the AIDS epidemic and the quality of health care provided to persons with AIDS has been extensively documented (Shilts, 1987a). AHB has often been targeted as a major factor underlying the slow response by the public and by the Federal government to the concerns of AIDS patients (Herek and Glunt, 1988). At various times, both the Center for Disease Control and the United States Senate have withheld support of potentially life-saving preventive education programs that explicitly described "safer sex" practices. In the language of the twice-endorsed Helms amendment, such materials could not be supported because of the danger that they might "promote or encourage, directly or indirectly, homosexual activities" (Herek and Glunt, 1988, p. 886). In 1988, the chairman of the President's Commission on AIDS identified fear of discrimination as "the most significant obstacle to progress" against the disease's spread (Blendon and Donelan, 1988, p. 1022).

As in the general public, fear and antipathy toward persons with AIDS have found their way into medicine and the mental health professions. One author has observed that "despite the opportunity of helpful intervention, palliation, and prevention in the form of psychological counseling, specialized services for AIDS patients and individuals-at-risk have met with resistance within psychiatry" (Seeman, 1989, p. 17).

Personal sentiment against AIDS patients may also act within individual clinical encounters, limiting the empathy and attention that HIV-positive patients receive and impairing the quality of their care. A number of studies have sought to examine the extent to which bias enters into the treatment of gay patients and patients with AIDS. Most of these efforts have used written surveys or fictional clinical vignettes to assess the attitudes and practices of clinicians from a variety of disciplines and levels of training. Investigators have used their results to make inferences about the actual clinical care AIDS patients receive. Collectively, this work suggests that health care professionals have more negative views of gay men and patients with AIDS than of other patients, with bias against gay men a principal determinant of AIDS bias.

The studies indicate that these views are present to a similar degree in all health care professions, including the mental health professions, and may be shaped by culture and personal exposure to such patients. Each study, whether the population surveyed consisted of physicians, medical students, nurses, or other hospital employees, showed a significant positive correlation between measured AHB and negative attitudes toward AIDS patients. Further, they suggest that such bias may impair the care AIDS patients receive through clinicians' lack of empathy or their refusal to treat HIV-positive patients (O'Donnell et al., 1987; D'Augilli, 1989; Henry, Campbell, and Willinbring, 1990).

For example, two studies, by Douglas et al. (1985) and by Wallack (1989), looked at attitudes among house staff and nurses in New York City hospitals. Douglas, Kalman, and Kalman (1985), using a standardized measure of attitudes toward gays (the Index of Homophobia [IHP]), a demographic questionnaire, and a series of eight questions regarding homosexuality and AIDS, surveyed more than 100 nurses and house officers at New York Hospital. The sample scored within the homophobic range of the IHP, and one third reported feeling "more negatively about homosexuality since the emergence of the AIDS crisis" (p. 1311). Nine per cent of respondents agreed with the statement that "[h]omosexuals who contract AIDS are getting what they deserve," calling into question the ability of some caregivers to treat AIDS patients sympathetically.

In a similar survey of nurses and house officers at New York's Beth Israel Medical Center, Wallack (1989) found that, in addition to a significant fear of acquiring AIDS, AHB was pronounced among the sampled caregivers. Almost half of those surveyed expressed anger at gays and associated the AIDS epidemic with homosexual promiscuity. This perceived etiological linkage fueled AHB. An impressive 18% of doctors and 33% of nurses agreed that "homosexual men afflicted with AIDS have only themselves to blame" (p. 508).

These findings are supported by the work of Smith et al. (1993), who surveyed 260 physicians and 240 other employees at a tertiary-care teaching hospital in Georgia. Negative attitudes toward AIDS patients were common among the clinical and nonclinical employees: "Misinformation, aversion, fear, and lack of compassion were evidenced by a substantial proportion of the respondents, particularly house staff" (p. 537). Surveying 161 students in medicine and nursing and paramedics, Royce and Birge (1987) measured fear of AIDS, empathy toward AIDS patients, and AHB with a 28-item questionnaire. The authors found that AHB was related to lack of empathy for AIDS patients and was a better predictor of fear of AIDS than age, sex, marital status, or discipline (p. 867). Similar attitudes have been demonstrated to lesser degrees among Canadian psychiatrists, psychiatry residents, and family practice residents (Chiamowitz, 1991). Studies have demonstrated comparable attitudes among American clinical psychologists and social workers (St. Lawrence et al., 1990; Crawford et al., 1994) and among Australian health care professionals (Hunter and Ross, 1991). A number of research teams have investigated the association of AHB and AIDS bias among health care workers. Each study, whether the population surveyed consisted of nurses, medical students, physicians, or other hospital employees, showed a significant positive correlation between measured AHB and negative attitudes toward AIDS patients (O'Donnell et al., 1987; D'Augilli, 1989; Henry et al., 1990).

While clearly documenting the presence of homophobia and AIDS bias among clinicians, these attitude surveys are limited in that they rely on retrospective self-report rather than on objective measurement of attitudes expressed in the clinical settings. Responses may be skewed toward views considered favorable or acceptable by clinicians. As health care professions generally subscribe to the importance of unbiased treatment for all patients, one would expect these surveys to underrepresent negative attitudes. Conversely, when one is faced with an actual patient, clinician empathy may temper the negative responses elicited by abstract questionnaires.

Studies using vignettes have attempted to predict more closely the response of clinicians to actual patients. Subjects in these studies are presented with fictional case vignettes differing only with respect to the diagnosis (AIDS or not AIDS) and sexual orientation of the patient described. Subjects then respond to a series of questions designed to assess their attitudes towards the patient. In these studies the use of non-AIDS and nongay patient vignettes controls for self-report bias, while the patient simulation allows for a closer assessment of the clinician's approach to actual patients. Their results confirm survey findings of clinician and trainee bias against gay men and AIDS status.

Kelly et al. (1987), for example, presented 119 medical students at the University of Mississippi with one of four case vignettes describing a male patient named Mark. The vignettes differed only in the illness attributed to the patient (he had either AIDS or leukemia) and his sexual orientation (his partner was named either Robert or Roberta). The students were then asked to fill out a questionnaire measuring their general attitudes toward the patient, their willingness to interact with him in a number of settings, and their sense of the patient's personal qualities. Overall, respondents rated the patient suffering from AIDS as more responsible for his illness, more deserving of what had happened to him, more deserving to die, and more deserving to lose his job than when he was described as having leukemia. The students were more willing to talk to the leukemic patient than to the AIDS patient.

Furthermore, the authors report, "Regardless of which disease was involved, the homosexual patients were viewed as being more responsible for their illness . . . more dangerous to others . . . and suffering less pain than the heterosexual patients" (p. 553). Those reading the case of a gay patient rated him as less attractive, less intelligent, less likable, and less truthful than the heterosexual patient. "In all areas," the authors conclude, "the students were less willing to interact, even in the most casual manner, with an individual identified as homosexual" (p. 554).

Although this section has explored the positive correlation between AHB and bias against persons with AIDS, it should be noted that in some instances attitudes toward the AIDS epidemic have correlated with more positive attitudes toward gay men. For example, the St. Lawrence et al. (1990) study of 126 practicing psychologists found that subjects rated the AIDS patient more negatively than the leukemic patient; however, respondents revealed more positive attitudes toward the gay patient than toward the identically described heterosexual patient.

Fear of Contagion as a Source of Bias

The sources of negative attitudes toward AIDS patients delineated earlier receive some empirical support in the literature. In particular, researchers examining the presence of fear of contagion and AHB have shown both to be positively correlated with AIDS bias.

Fear of contagion (assessed through written questionnaires as well as personal interviews) has been shown to be prominent among physicians and nurses despite data that HIV is not spread through ordinary contact in clinical practice (Wallack, 1989; Epstein et al., 1993). Importantly, where such correlations could be measured, those groups expressing greater fear of acquiring AIDS at work also expressed greater bias against gay men and against patients with AIDS (Wallack, 1989; Blumenfield et al., 1991). Simon et al. (1991), in their assessment of medical student attitudes toward HIV-positive patients, found that homophobia, but not perceived risk of infection, was negatively correlated with intention to treat HIV-positive patients.

Cultural Aspects of AHB and Fear of HIV in Health Workers

A few studies measuring attitudes across different groups have pointed to the effects of culture and experience in shaping practitioner bias. Providing the most detailed assessment of the interaction between ethnicity and attitude, Wallack's 1989 survey of New York physicians and nurses found that in both disciplines nonwhite respondents (listed as Black, Hispanic, and Asian) were more uncomfortable with gay patients and more fearful of acquiring AIDS. Among nurses, Asians showed significantly less empathy for gay men with AIDS than did other minority respondents, whereas Black nurses showed the least bias of the three nonwhite groups. Jewish respondents, irrespective of discipline, were more likely to be comfortable treating gay patients than were Protestants or Catholics. This investigation did not control for variables related to social class, however, and the differences between groups might not have been entirely due to the influence of ethnicity.

Like ethnicity, nationality of caregivers may affect AIDS bias. A 1992 survey of medical house staff in the United States, Canada, and France showed significantly greater reluctance to treat AIDS patients among Americans (23% would refuse care) than among Canadian and French respondents (14% and 4%, respectively, would refuse care (Shapiro et al., 1992, p. 510).

The literature offers no conclusive data regarding the relative distribution of AIDS bias and homophobia (AHB) among different professions. Both Wallack (1989) and Douglas et al. (1985) showed a trend toward greater AHB and AIDS bias among nurses than among residents; the variable of profession was, however, not considered independent of such other variables as education, age, gender, ethnicity, religion, and years of experience, variables which differed significantly between the two groups. Smith et al. (1993) found negative attitudes sampled across all physicians and other hospital employees to be higher among house staff than among senior physicians. Chiamowitz (1991), however, found that in a Canadian teaching hospital residents in psychiatry and family practice were more willing to treat AIDS patients than were psychiatric faculty members. Crawford et al. (1991) reported no difference in attitudes between clinical psychologists and social workers in reactions to case vignettes.

Those studies which evaluated bias among professionals at a similar level of training suggest that greater experience with AIDS patients may be correlated with less bias (e.g., Dow and Knox, 1991). For example, Bresolin et al. (1990) found that among 500 primary-care physicians interviewed by telephone, support for mandatory testing and contact tracing, often associated with less empathy for AIDS patients, decreased as contact with AIDS patients increased. While these findings may suggest that increased contact with AIDS patients leads to more favorable attitudes, they may also simply indicate that those with less bias are more willing to have contact with AIDS patients.

Impact of AHB on Patient Care

The studies just outlined indicate that many clinicians approach AIDS patients with less empathy than they show other patients. Just as such bias has led to discriminatory behaviors in other arenas, such as housing and employment, one would suspect that negative attitudes among clinicians might lead to a diminution of quality in health care for HIV-positive individuals. No studies directly supporting such a conclusion are yet available in the medical and psychological literature. The surveys' clear demonstration of AIDS bias, for example, need not necessarily translate into poor care, as clinicians' behavior may be guided more by professional ideals than by personal biases in the treatment of patients. Yet the literature does provide indirect evidence that negative views of AIDS patients and gay men have translated into inferior care for HIV-positive patients. Such evidence comes from clinicians' anecdotal reports that they have observed discrimination by others and from their statements that they themselves discriminate against patients with AIDS.

When questioned, survey respondents frequently reported that patients with AIDS received substandard care within their institution. Over half of those polled by Chiamowitz (1991) and approximately one-third of Douglas et al.'s (1985) respondents felt that hospitalized AIDS patients received care inferior to that offered patients with other illnesses. Thirty-nine per cent of medical house officers surveyed throughout the United States reported that an HIV-positive patient under their care had been refused treatment by a surgeon, 19% by a medical specialist (Shapiro et al., 1992, p. 510).

In his survey of nurses and house officers at New York's Beth Israel Medical Center, Wallack (1989) found more direct support for the hypothesis that bias and fear among health workers may affect AIDS patients' care: over half of those responding reported that they tend to avoid performing procedures on AIDS patients because of fear of contagion. Similarly, Blumenfeld et al. (1991) found that of over 200 medical-surgical nurses at a Westchester hospital 42% stated that they were unwilling to care for AIDS patients. A 1991 survey of Missouri physicians revealed that less than half the respondents were willing to treat HIV-positive patients and even fewer would take on a patient with AIDS (Baumgartner, Hangar-Mace, and Dabney, 1991), while 40% of physicians in North Carolina reported refusing or referring new HIV-positive patients elsewhere (Weinberger et al., 1992).

Implications for the Clinician

In their work with other caregivers, mental health professionals have the opportunity to ameliorate the negative reactions that HIV-positive patients encounter in medical settings. Those who work in the consult-liaison area, in particular, may help other members of the treatment team modify their reactions to patients, clearing the way for more consistent and compassionate care (Wallack, 1989). By taking an active role in the education, training, and supervision of future caregivers, teachers may help to counter the bias that some suggest correlates with less exposure to gay and HIV-positive patients and their concerns (Royse and Birge, 1987; Crawford et al., 1991). In their work with HIV-positive patients, psychiatrists may pay particular attention to the debilitating effects of widespread antipathy on patients.

The stigmatization that all HIV-positive patients live with compounds the psychological morbidity of the disorder. Patients risk rejection by important others when their illness is disclosed, yet the concealment of a positive serostatus can also result in profound isolation. To the gay man already conflicted about his sexual orientation, a diagnosis of HIV-positivity may seem a retribution, fortifying his own feelings of guilt. For some heterosexual patients, the disorder, even if not acquired sexually, brings with it unsettling implications regarding the patients' sexual orientation, because it is felt to link them with a community they may not view favorably.

Shame, a natural sequel of perceiving oneself as a member of a hated group, contributes significantly to the emotional burden of HIV infection (Schaffner, 1986, 1990, 1993, 1996).

Conclusion

A number of scholars have examined the sources for AIDS' stigmatization (Brandt, 1987; Sontag, 1988; Herek and Glunt, 1988; Seeman, 1989). Among those sources postulated are the characteristics of the disease itself and the chance associations made to its mode of transmission and its distribution.

AIDS belongs to a broad category of diseases that Goffman (1963) has termed "abominations of the body" (p. 4). The dramatic physical deterioration that AIDS wreaks causes its sufferers to have physical anomalies that challenge notions of bodily integrity and arouse fear and disgust in those who encounter them (Douglas, 1966). As Sontag (1988) observes, those diseases which "transform the body into something alienating" have historically been the most dreaded (p. 89).

The fatality of the illness brings observers face-to-face with the reality of death, provoking in them what Schutz has termed the "fundamental anxiety" (quoted in Herek and Glunt, 1988). Healthy people distance themselves from death by defining terminal illness as an affliction of others. According to Schutz, one pragmatic objective of daily life is to construct experiences that avoid this fundamental anxiety. AIDS-related stigmatization represents such a construction.

The communicability of the disease undermines the capacity of the uninfected to affirm their sense of safety from its misfortunes, thus elevating anxiety and, consequently, antipathy. Interestingly, those who overestimate their own vulnerability to contagion (such as through casual contact) are also likely to focus on infection as being the outcome of a willful act. These contradictory notions of easy communicability and easy avoidance of infection (through control of one's appetites for sex or drugs) together contribute to the social opprobrium directed toward persons with AIDS (Herek and Glunt, 1988; Seeman, 1989). As a sexually transmitted disease, AIDS collects further discredit as it simultaneously connotes sexual activity and dictates the need to curb it, two notions similarly troublesome to the American mind.

Most significant for the purposes of this report, however, is the role of AIDS' association with already stigmatized groups, particularly homosexual males, in creating negative public attitudes toward it. Like leprosy, HIV came to be hated not only for its feared effects but also because of the stigma of those who most heavily bore them.

The relationship between homosexuality and AIDS has been one of mutually reinforcing stigma. Its early association with male homosexual behavior played an important role in the development of widespread fear of and contempt for HIV and those it infected. The outbreak of a fatal and communicable illness among the gay community deepened Americans' long-standing antihomosexual bias. One cannot understand the full scope of present day AHB without taking into account the effect of AIDS on the public imagination. The disease has flushed into open view covert hostilities toward gays held both by health professionals and by the lay public, while simultaneously exacerbating those views. Linked through an accident of social history, AHB and fear of AIDS have met in a synergy of stigma with consequent adverse effects on the physical and mental health of gays and persons with AIDS alike.

Changes have occurred in the attitudes of mental health professionals since the outbreak of the AIDS epidemic. There is a lessening of AHB, evidenced by the acceptance of openly gay and lesbian candidates in psychiatric, psychological, and other training institutes. Openly gay and lesbian mental health workers are more outspoken as individuals and in gay and lesbian professional organizations. The development of new drugs to prolong and improve the lives of those with HIV to some extent may diminish fear of AIDS. More hopeful treatments for HIV may mutually reinforce more positive attitudes toward gay men.

6 CONCLUSION

In this report, the Committee on Human Sexuality has tried to identify the essential aspects of antihomosexual bias. Increased familiarity with the repercussions of AHB should enable clinicians to feel more comfortable working with lesbian and gay patients. This heightened insight, in turn, will counteract the tendency to dehumanize these patients and will allow therapists to relate to them in a caring, nonjudgmental way. Therapists will be able to engage in more constructive therapeutic dialogue, and patients and therapists are likely to emerge from the treatment situation with a greater sense of accomplishment and satisfaction. Patients will benefit from such changes through improved quality of care; some lesbian and gay patients actually avoided psychotherapy in recent years because of the profession's reputation for AHB.

The changes following "gay liberation" and the AIDS epidemic have come so rapidly that many older lesbians and gay men have been surpised and overwhelmed by them, whereas younger lesbians and gay men seem often to take those changes for granted. It is likely that mental health professionals as a group will follow a similar pattern.

In the last quarter century, the curricula in educational and psychotherapy training institutions have come to include courses on gay and lesbian psychotherapy and treatment. Many professional organizations, including the American Psychiatric Association, the American Psychological Association, the American Psychoanalytic Association, the American Academy of Psychoanalysis, the National Association of Social Workers, and the American Orthopsychiatric Association, have passed declarations of policy barring all discrimination against admission and training of mental health professionals on the basis of sexual orientation.

As a consequence, it is likely that there will be more openly identified lesbian and gay clinicians to treat lesbian and gay patients. Concurrently, there is also a rapidly developing body of knowledge concerning the intricacies of transference and countertransference problems when the sexual orientation of the therapist is not openly stated or is different from that of the patient. Today, as a result of antidiscrimination policy and legislation, lesbian and gay therapists, as well as patients, are less reluctant to disclose their sexual orientation to their colleagues and employers. These social changes have introduced a note of caution in the open expression of AHB or actions on the part of authorities.

It is hoped that this Committee report will be both interesting and of practical use to those who read it. Above all, it is hoped that it will stimulate all psychotherapists to become curious about their own unconscious AHB, to familiarize themselves with its manifestations, and to do their best to prevent it from unintentionally harming their patients.

References

Abelove, H. (1985), Freud, male homosexuality, and the Americans. In *The Lesbian and Gay Studies Reader*, ed. H. Abelove, M. A. Barale & D. Halperin. New York: Routledge, 1993, pp. 381–393.

Abelove, H., Barale, M. A. & Halperin, D., eds. (1993), *The Lesbian and Gay Studies Reader*. New York: Routledge.

Achtenberg, R. (1987), *Sexual Orientation and the Law*. New York: Clark Boardman.

Acton, W. (1865), *The Functions and Disorders of the Reproductive System*. London: J. & A. Churchill.

American Academy of Pediatrics Committee on Adolescence (1993), Homosexuality and adolescence. *Pediat.*, 92:631–634.

American Association of Directors of Psychiatric Residency Training (1978), second annual questionnaire, October.

American Psychiatric Association (1952), *Diagnostic and Statistical Manual of Mental Disorders, 1st Edition*. Washington, DC: American Psychiatric Press.

American Psychiatric Association (1968), *Diagnostic and Statistical Manual of Mental Disorders, 2nd Edition*. Washington, DC: American Psychiatric Press.

American Psychiatric Association (1980), *Diagnostic and Statistical Manual of Mental Disorders, 3rd Edition*. Washington, DC: American Psychiatric Press.

American Psychiatric Association (1987), *Diagnostic and Statistical Manual of Mental Disorders, 3rd Edition-Revised*. Washington, DC: American Psychiatric Press.

American Psychiatric Association (1993), *The Principles of Medical Ethics: With Annotations Especially Applicable to Psychiatry*. Washington, DC: American Psychiatric Press.

American Psychoanalytic Association (1996), The American's

antidiscrimination policy on homosexuality. *Amer. Psychoanal.*, 30(3):21.
Appeal in Pima City Juvenile Action 727 P. 2d 830, 835 (1986).
Baehr v. Lewin, 852 P.2d 44 (Haw. 1993).
Baehr v. Miike, State of Hawaii, First Circuit, West Law 694235 (1996).
Baumeyer, F. (1956), The Schreber case. *Internat. J. Psycho-Anal.,* 37:61-74.
Baumgartner, T. F., Haagar-Mace, L., & Dabney, S. (1991), HIV/AIDS in Missouri: An assessment of physician attitudes and practices. *Missouri Med.,* 88:28-32.
Bayer, R. (1981), *Homosexuality and American Psychiatry: The Politics of Diagnosis.* New York: Basic Books.
Bell, A. & Weinberg, M. (1978), *Homosexualities: A Study of Diversity Among Men and Women.* New York: Simon & Schuster.
Bell, A., Weinberg, M. & Hammersmith S. (1981), *Sexual Preference: Its Development in Men and Women.* Bloomington: Indiana University Press.
Bergler, E. (1944), Eight prerequisites for psychoanalytic treatment of homosexuality. *Psychoanal. Rev.,* 31:253-286.
Bergler, E. (1951), *Counterfeit Sex: Homosexuality, Impotence, Frigidity.* New York: Grune & Stratton.
Bergler, E. (1956), *Homosexuality: Disease or Way of Life.* New York: Hill & Wang.
Berzon, B. (1988), *Permanent Partners: Building Gay and Lesbian Relationships That Last.* New York: Dutton.
Bezio v. Patenaude, 381 Mass. 563, 576-577, 410 N.E. 2nd 1207 (Mass S.J.C. 1980).
Bieber, I., Dain, H., Dince, P., Drellich, M., Grand, H., Gundlach, R., Kremer, M., Rifkin, A., Wilbur, C. & Bieber T. (1962), *Homosexuality: A Psychoanalytic Study.* New York: Basic Books.
Blechner, M. (1993), Homophobia in psychoanalytic writing and practice. *Psychoanal. Dial.,* 3:627-637.
Blendon, R. J. & Donelan, K. (1988), Discrimination against people with AIDS. *New Engl. J. Med.,* 319:1022-1026.
Blumenfield, M., Milazzo, J., Wormser, G. P. & Smith, P. J. (1991), Reluctance to care for patients with AIDS. *Gen. Hosp. Psychiat.,* 13:410.
Blumstein, P. & Schwartz, P. (1983), *American Couples: Money, Work, Sex.* New York: William Morris.
Bonauto, M. (1993), *National Overview of Lesbian, Gay and Other*

Nontraditional Domestic Relations and Probate Law. Boston, MA: GLAD.
Boswell, J. (1980), *Christianity, Social Tolerance and Homosexuality.* Chicago: University of Chicago Press.
Boswell, J. (1994), *Same-Sex Unions in Premodern Europe.* New York: Villard Books.
Bottoms v. Bottoms, 249 VA 410, 418–420 (1995).
Bowers v. Hardwick, (1986) 487 US 186.
Bozett, F. W. (1987), Children of gay fathers. In *Gay and Lesbian Parents,* ed. F. W. Bozett. New York: Praeger, pp. 39–57.
Brandt, A. M. (1987), *No Magic Bullet: A Social History of Venereal Disease in the United States Since 1880, with a New Chapter on AIDS.* New York: Oxford University Press.
Bresolin, L. B., Rinaldi, R. C., Henning, J. J., Harvey, L. K., Hendee, W. R. & Schwarz, M. R. (1990), Attitudes of US primary care physicians about HIV disease and AIDS. *AIDS Care,* 2:117–125.
Brown, L. S. (1996), Ethical concerns with sexual minority patients. In *Textbook of Homosexuality and Mental Health,* ed. R. Cabaj & T. Stein. Washington, DC: American Psychiatric Press, pp. 897–916.
Bullough, V. (1979), *Homosexuality: A History.* New York: Meridian.
Butler, J. (1990), *Gender Trouble: Feminism and the Subversion of Identity.* New York: Routledge.
Buxton, A. (1994), *The Other Side of the Closet: The Coming-Out Crisis for Straight Spouses and Families,* 2nd ed. New York: Wiley.
Cabaj, R. & Stein, T., eds. (1996), *Textbook of Homosexuality and Mental Health.* Washington, DC: American Psychiatric Press.
Cabaj, R. (1988), Gay and lesbian couples: Lessons on human intimacy. *Psychiat. Annals,* 18:21–25.
Cabalquinto v. Cabalquinto, 718 P.2d 7 (1986).
Cameron, N. (1967), Paranoid reaction. In *Comprehensive Textbook of Psychiatry,* ed. A. M. Freedman & H. I. Kaplan. Baltimore, MD: Williams & Wilkins.
Carl, D. (1990), *Counseling Same-Sex Couples.* New York: Norton.
Chiamowitz, G. A. (1991), Homophobia among psychiatric residents, family practice residents and psychiatric faculty. *Canad. J. Psychiat.,* 36:206–209 .
Chodorow, N. (1978), *The Reproduction of Mothering.* Berkeley: University of California Press.
Clark, T. R. (1975), Homosexuality and psychopathology in nonpatient males. *Amer. J. Psychoanal.,* 35:163–168.

Coates, S., Friedman, R. C. & Wolfe, S. (1991), The etiology of boyhood gender identity disorder: A model for integrating temperament, development, and psychodynamics. *Psychoanal. Dial.*, 1:481–523.
Colasanto, D. (1989), Gay rights support has grown since 1982, Gallup Poll finds. *San Francisco Chronicle*, October 25, p. A21.
Cort, J. & Corlevale, E. (1982), Murder in Maine renews interest in rights bill. *The Advocate*, 42(9/4):12, 13.
Crawford, I., Humfleet, G., Ribordy, S. C., Ho, F. C. & Vickers, V. L. (1991), Stigmatization of AIDS patients by metal health professionals. *Profess. Psychol. Res. & Pract.*, 22:357–361.
D'Augelli, A. R. (1989), AIDS fears and homophobia among rural nursing personnel, *AIDS Ed. & Prev.* 1:277–284.
D'Augelli, A. R. & Patterson, C. (1995), *Lesbian, Gay and Bisexual Identities Over the Lifespan.* New York: Oxford University Press.
Davison, G. C. & Wilson, G. T. (1974), Goals and strategies in behavioral treatment of homosexual pedophilia: Comments on a case study. *J. Abnorm. Psychol.*, 83:196–198.
De Cecco, J., ed. (1985), *Bashers, Baiters & Bigots: Homophobia in American Society.* New York: Harrington Park Press.
De Cecco, J., ed. (1988), *Gay Relationships.* New York: Harrington Park Press.
De Cecco, J. & Parker, D., eds. (1995), *Sex, Cells and Same-Sex Desire: The Biology of Sexual Preference.* New York: Harrington Park Press.
Defense of Marriage Act, 104 Public Law 199, 110 Stat. 2419 (1996).
Domenici, T. & Lesser, R., eds. (1995) *Disorienting Sexuality: Psychoanalytic Reappraisals of Sexual Identities.* New York: Routledge.
Douglas, C. J., Kalman, C. M. & Kalman, T. P. (1985), Homophobia among physicians and nurses: An empirical study. *Hosp. Comm. Psychiat.*, 36:1309–1311.
Douglas, M. (1966), *Purity and Danger: An Analysis of the Concepts of Pollution and Taboo.* London: Routledge & Kegan Paul.
Dow, M. G. & Knox, M. D. (1991), Mental health and substance abuse staff: HIV/AIDS knowledge and attitudes. *AIDS Care*, 3:75–87.
Downey, J. & Friedman, R. C. (1995), Internalized homophobia in lesbian relationships. *J. Amer. Acad. Psychoanal.*, 23: 435–447.
Downey, J. & Friedman, R. C. (1996), The negative therapeutic reaction and self-hatred in gay and lesbian patients. In *Homo-*

sexuality and Mental Health: A Comprehensive Textbook, ed. R. Cabaj & T. Stein. Washington, DC: American Psychiatric Press, pp. 471-484.

Drescher, J. (1995), Anti-homosexual bias in training. In *Disorienting Sexualities*, ed. T. Domenici & R. Lesser. New York: Routledge, pp. 227-241.

Drescher, J. (1996a), Psychoanalytic subjectivity and male homosexuality. In *Textbook of Homosexuality and Mental Health*, ed. R. Cabaj & T. Stein. Washington, DC: American Psychiatric Press, pp. 173-189.

Drescher, J. (1996b), A discussion across sexual orientation and gender boundaries: Reflections of a gay male analyst to a heterosexual female analyst. *Gender & Psychoanal.*, 1(2):223-237.

Drescher, J. (1996c), Across the great divide: Gender panic in the psychoanalytic dyad. *Psychoanal. & Psychother.*, 13:174-186.

Drescher, J. (1997), From preoedipal to postmodern: Changing psychoanalytic attitudes toward homosexuality. *Gender & Psychoanal.*, 2:203-216.

Drescher, J. (1998a), Contemporary psychoanalytic psychotherapy with gay men: With a commentary on reparative therapy of homosexuality. *J. Gay & Lesbian Psychother.*, 2(4):51-74

Drescher, J. (1998b), *Psychoanalytic Therapy and the Gay Man*. Hillsdale, NJ: The Analytic Press.

Duberman, M. (1986), *About Time: Exploring the Gay Past*. New York: Sea Horse.

Duberman, M. (1991), *Cures: A Gay Man's Odyssey*. New York: Dutton.

Dunlap, D. (1995), Shameless homophobia and the "Jenny Jones" murder. *The New York Times*, March 19.

Ellis, H. (1938), *Psychology of Sex*. New York: Harcourt Brace Jovanovich.

England v. State of Texas WL 30503 (1993).

Epstein, R. M., Christie, M., Frankel, R., Rousseau, S., Shields, C. & Suchman, A. L. (1993), Understanding fear of contagion among physicians who care for HIV patients. *Fam. Med.*, 25:264-268.

Erikson, E. H. (1959), The problem of ego identity. In *Identity and the Life Cycle*. New York: International Universities Press, pp. 101-164.

Falco, K. (1996), Psychotherapy with women who love women. In: *Textbook of Homosexuality and Mental Health*, ed. R. Cabaj & T. Stein. Washington, DC: American Psychiatric Press, pp. 397-412.

REFERENCES

Falk P. (1989), Lesbian mothers: Psychological assumptions in family law. *Amer. Psychol.*, 44:941–947.
Fenichel, O. (1945), *The Psychoanalytic Theory of Neurosis*. New York: Norton.
Fine, G. A. (1987), *With the Boys: Little League Baseball and Preadolescent Culture*. Chicago: University of Chicago Press.
Fisher, S. & Greenberg, R. P. (1985), *The Scientific Credibility of Freud's Theories and Therapy*. New York: Columbia University Press.
Ford, C. & Beach, F. (1951), *Patterns of Sexual Behavior*. New York: Harper.
Fort, J., Steiner, C. M. & Conrad, F. (1971), Attitudes of mental health professionals toward homosexuality and its treatment. *Psychol. Rep.*, 29:347–350.
Foucault, M. (1978), *The History of Sexuality, Volume I, An Introduction*. New York: Vintage, 1980.
Freud, S. (1905), Three essays on the theory of sexuality. *Standard Edition*, 7:123–246. London: Hogarth Press, 1953.
Freud, S. (1910), Leonardo da Vinci and a memory of his childhood. *Standard Edition*, 11:59–138. London: Hogarth Press, 1957.
Freud, S. (1911), Psycho-analytic notes on an autobiographical account of a case of paranoia. *Standard Edition*, 12:1–82. London: Hogarth Press, 1958.
Freud, S. (1912), Recommendations to physicians practicing psychoanalysis. *Standard Edition*, 12:109–120. London: Hogarth Press, 1958.
Freud, S. (1920), The psychogenesis of a case of homosexuality in a woman. *Standard Edition*, 18:221–232. London: Hogarth Press, 1955.
Freud, S. (1933), New introductory lectures on psycho-analysis. *Standard Edition*, 22:1–182. London: Hogarth Press, 1964.
Freud, S. (1937), Analysis terminable and interminable. *Standard Edition*, 22:209–253. London: Hogarth Press, 1964.
Friedman, R. C. (1983), Book review: *Homosexuality* by C. W. Socarides. *J. Amer. Psychoanal. Assn.*, 31:316–323.
Friedman, R. C. (1988), *Male Homosexuality: A Contemporary Psychoanalytic Perspective*. New Haven, CT: Yale University Press.
Friedman, R. C. & Downey, J. (1993a), Neurobiology and sexual orientation: Current relationships. *J. Neuropsychiat. Clin. Neurosci.*, 5:131–153.
Friedman, R. C. & Downey, J. (1993b), Psychoanalysis, psychobiology, and homosexuality. *J. Amer. Psychoanal. Assn.*, 41:1159–1198.

Friedman, R. C. & Downey, J. (1994), Homosexuality. *New Engl. J. Med.*, 331:923–930.

Friedman, R. C. & Downey, J. (1995a), Biology and the Oedipus complex. *Psychoanal. Quart.*, 64:234–264.

Friedman, R. C. & Downey, J. (1995b), Internalized homophobia and the negative therapeutic reaction. *J. Amer. Acad. Psychoanal.*, 23:99–113.

Friedman, R. C. & Lilling, A. (1996), An empirical study of the beliefs of psychoanalysts about scientific and clinical dimensions of male homosexuality. *J. Homosex.*, 32(2):79–89.

Frommer, M. S. (1995), Countertransference obscurity in the treatment of homosexual patients. In: *Disorienting Sexualities*, ed. T. Domenici & R. Lesser. New York: Routledge, pp. 65–82.

Gay, P. (1988), *Freud: A Life for Our Time*. New York: Norton.

Gilligan, C. (1982), *In a Different Voice*. Cambridge, MA: Harvard University Press.

Goffman, E. (1963), *Stigma: Notes on the Management of Spoiled Identity*. Englewood Cliffs, NJ: Prentice-Hall.

Golombok, S., Spencer, A. & Rutter, M. (1983), Children in lesbian and single-parent households: Psychosexual and psychiatric appraisal. *J. Child. Psychol. Psychiat.*, 24:551–572.

Gomes, P. J. (1996). *The Good Book: Reading the Bible with Mind and Heart*. New York: Avon.

Gonsiorek, J. C. (1991), The empirical basis for the demise of the illness model of homosexuality. In *Homosexuality: Research Implications for Public Policy*, ed. J. D. Gonsiorek & J. D. Weinrich. Newbury Park, CA: Sage, pp. 115–137.

Gonsiorek, J. C. & Weinrich, J. D., eds. (1991), *Homosexuality: Research Implications for Public Policy*. Newbury Park, CA: Sage.

Gottman, J. S. (1990), Children of lesbian and gay parents. In *Homosexuality and Family Relations*, ed. F. W. Bozett & M. B. Susman. New York: Harrington Park Press, pp. 177–196.

Green, G. D. & Bozett, F. W. (1991), Lesbian mothers and gay fathers. In *Homosexuality: Research Implications for Public Policy*, ed. J. C. Gonsiorek & J. D. Weinrich. Newbury Park, CA: Sage, pp. 197–214.

Green, R. (1985), Gender identity in childhood and later sexual orientation: Follow-up of 78 males. *Amer. J. Psychiat.*, 142:339–341.

Green, R. (1987), *The "Sissy Boy Syndrome" and the Development of Homosexuality*. New Haven, CT: Yale University Press.

Green, R., Mandel, J. B., Hotvedt, M. E., Gray, J. & Smith, L. (1986),

REFERENCES

Lesbian mothers and their children: A comparison with solo parent heterosexual mothers and their children. *Arch. Sex. Behav.*, 15:167–184.

Greenberg, D. (1988), *The Construction of Homosexuality*. Chicago: University of Chicago Press.

Greenson, R. R. (1968), Disidentifying from mother. *Internat. J. Psycho-Anal.*, 49:370–374.

Group for the Advancement of Psychiatry (1950a), *Psychiatrically Deviated Sex Offenders*, Report No. 9. Topeka, KS: GAP.

Group for the Advancement of Psychiatry (1950b), *The Social Responsibility of Psychiatry: A Statement of Orientation*, Report No. 13. Topeka, KS: GAP.

Group for the Advancement of Psychiatry (1955), *Homosexuality with Particular Emphasis on This Problem in Governmental Agencies*, Report No. 30. Topeka, KS: GAP.

Group for the Advancement of Psychiatry (1957), *The Psychiatric Aspects of School Desegregation*, Report No. 37. Chicago: Aldine.

Group for the Advancement of Psychiatry (1960), *Sex and the College Student*, Report No. 60. Topeka, KS: GAP.

Group for the Advancement of Psychiatry (1973), *Assessment of Sexual Function: A Guide to Interviewing*, Report No. 88. New York: GAP.

Group for the Advancement of Psychiatry (1975), *The Educated Woman: Prospects and Problems*, Report No. 92. New York: GAP.

Group for the Advancement of Psychiatry (1977), *Psychiatry and Sex Psychopath Legislation: The 30's to the 80's*, Report No. 98. New York: GAP.

Group for the Advancement of Psychiatry (1986), *Crises of Adolescence: Teenage Pregnancy: Impact on Adolescent Development*, Report No. 118. New York: Brunner/Mazel.

Group for the Advancement of Psychiatry (1990), *Psychotherapy with College Students*, Report No. 130. New York: Brunner/Mazel.

Hancock, K. A. (1995), Psychotherapy with lesbians and gay men. In *Lesbian, Gay and Bisexual Identities Over the Lifespan*, ed. A. R. D'Augelli & C. J. Patterson. New York: Oxford University Press, pp. 398–432.

Hanley-Hackenbruck, P. (1993), Working with lesbians in psychotherapy. *Rev. Psychiat.*, 12:59–83.

Harris, A. (1991), Gender as contradiction. *Psychoanal. Dial.*, 1:197–224.

REFERENCES

Harvard Law Review (1985), The constitutional status of sexual orientation: Homosexuality as a suspect classification. *Harvard Law Rev.*, 98:1285–1302.

Harvey, J. (1987), *The Homosexual Person: New Thinking in Pastoral Care.* San Francisco, CA: Ignatius.

Hatterer, L. (1970), *Changing Homosexuality in the Male.* New York: McGraw Hill.

Helminiak, D. (1994), *What the Bible Really Says About Homosexuality.* San Francisco, CA: Alamo Press.

Hendin, H. (1992), Suicide among homosexual youth. *Amer. J. Psychiat.*, 149:1416–1417.

Henry, K., Campbell, S. & Willinbring, K (1990), A cross-sectional analysis of variables impacting on AIDS-related knowledge, attitudes and behaviors among employees of a Minnesota teaching hospital. *AIDS Ed. & Prev.*, 2:36–47.

Herek, G. (1984), Beyond homophobia: A social psychological perspective on the attitudes towards lesbians and gay men. In *Bashers, Baiters & Bigots: Homophobia in American Society*, ed. J. DeCecco. New York: Harrington Park Press, 1985, pp. 1–21.

Herek, G. M. (1990), The context of anti-gay violence: Notes on cultural and psychological heterosexism. *J. Interpers. Viol.*, 5:316–333.

Herek, G. M. (1995), Psychological heterosexism in the United States. In *Lesbian, Gay and Bisexual Identities Over the Lifespan*, ed. A. R. D'Augelli & C. J. Patterson. Oxford, UK: Oxford University Press, pp. 321–346.

Herek, G. M. & Berrill, K., eds. (1990). Violence against lesbians and gay men: Issues for research, practice and policy. *J. Interpers. Viol.*, Special Issue 5(3).

Herek, G. M. & Berrill, K. (1992), *Hate Crimes: Confronting Violence Against Lesbians and Gay Men.* Newbury Park, CA: Sage.

Herek G. M. & Glunt, E. K. (1988), An epidemic of stigma: Public reactions to AIDS. *Amer. Psychol.*, 43:886–889.

Holt, R. R. (1989), *Freud Reappraised.* New York: Guilford Press.

Hooker, E. (1957), The adjustment of the male overt homosexual. In *The Problem of Homosexuality in Modern America*, ed. H. M. Ruitenbeck. New York: Dutton, 1963, pp. 141–161.

Hunter, C. E. & Ross, M. W. (1991), Determinants of health-care workers' attitudes toward people with AIDS. *J. Appl. Social Psychol.*, 21:947–956.

Hunter, N. (1991), Marriage, law, and gender: A feminist inquiry. *Law & Sexuality*, 1:9–30.

REFERENCES

Isay, R. (1989), *Being Homosexual: Gay Men and Their Development.* New York: Farrar, Straus & Giroux.

Isay, R. (1991), The homosexual analyst: Clinical considerations. *The Psychoanalytic Study of the Child,* 46:199–216. New Haven, CT: Yale University Press.

Isay, R. (1996), *Becoming Gay: The Journey to Self-Acceptance.* New York: Pantheon.

Jones, F. & Koshes, R. (1995), Homosexuality and the military. *Amer. J. Psychiat.,* 152:16–21.

Kelly, J. A., St. Lawrence, J. S. & Smith, S. Jr. (1987), Medical students' attitudes toward AIDS and homosexual patients. *J. Med. Ed.,* 62:549–556.

Kiersky, S. (1996), Exiled desire: The problem of reality in psychoanalysis and lesbian experience. *Psychoanal. & Psychother.,* 13:130–141.

Kinsey, A., Pomeroy, W. & Martin, C. (1948), *Sexual Behavior in the Human Male.* Philadelphia, PA: Saunders.

Kinsey, A., Pomeroy, W., Martin, C. & Gebhard, P. (1953), *Sexual Behavior in the Human Female.* Philadelphia, PA: Saunders.

Kirkpatrick, M. (1987), Clinical implications of lesbian mother studies. *J. Homosexual.,* 13:201–211.

Kirkpatrick, M. (1996), Lesbians as parents. In: *Textbook of Homosexuality and Mental Health,* ed. R. Cabaj & T. Stein. Washington, DC: American Psychiatric Press, pp. 353–370.

Kirkpatrick, M., Smith, C. & Roy, R. (1981), Lesbian mothers and their children: A comparative survey. *Amer. J. Orthopsychiat.,* 51:545–551.

Klaf, F. S. & Davis, C. A. (1960), Homosexuality and paranoid schizophrenia: a survey of 150 cases and controls. *Amer. J. Psychiat.,* 116:1070–1075.

Klassen, A. P., Williams, C. J. & Levitt, E. E. (1989), *Sex and Morality in the US* Middletown, CT: Wesleyan University Press.

Klein, H. R. & Horowitz, W. A. (1949), Psychosexual factors in the paranoid phenomena. *Amer. J. Psychiat.,* 105:697–701.

Kleinman A. (1988), *Illness Narratives: Suffering, Healing, and the Human Condition.* New York: Basic Books.

Klinger, R. L. & Stein, T. S. (1996), Impact of violence, childhood sexual abuse and domestic violence and abuse on lesbians, bisexuals and gay men. In *Textbook of Homosexuality and Mental Health,* ed. R. P. Cabaj & T. S. Stein. Washington, DC: American Psychiatric Press, pp. 801–818.

Krafft-Ebing, R. (1886), *Psychopathia Sexualis*, trans. H. Wedeck. New York: Putnam, 1965.

Kwawer, J. (1980), Transference and countertransference in homosexuality: Changing psychoanalytic views. *Amer. J. Pyschother.*, 34:72–80.

Lesser, R. (1993), A reconsideration of homosexual themes. *Psychoanal. Dial.*, 3:639–641.

Levenson, E. (1983), *The Ambiguity of Change.* New York: Basic Books.

Lewes, K. (1988), *Psychoanalysis and Male Homosexuality.* Northvale, NJ: Aronson, 1995.

Lief, H. (1977), Current thinking on homosexuality. *Med. Aspects Human Sexual.*, 11:110–111.

Lilling, A. & Friedman, R. C. (1995), Bias towards gay patients by psychoanalytic clinicians: An empirical investigation. *Arch. Sex. Behav.*, 24:563–570.

Magee, M. & Miller, D. (1995), Assaults and harassments: The violent acts of theorizing lesbian sexuality. Presented at panel "Psychoanalysis and Homosexuality: A Contemporary View," American Acad. Psychoanalysis, December 10.

Magee, M. & Miller, D. (1997), *Lesbian Lives: Psychoanalytic Narratives Old and New.* Hillsdale, NJ: The Analytic Press.

Marmor, J., ed. (1980), *Homosexual Behavior: A Modern Reappraisal.* New York: Basic Books.

McCrary, J. & Guitierrez, L. (1980), The homosexual person in the military and in national security employment. *J. Homosexual.*, 5:115–146.

McWhirter, D. & Mattison, A. (1984), *The Male Couple: How Relationships Develop.* Englewood Cliffs, NJ: Prentice-Hall.

McWhirter, D., Sanders, S. & Reinisch, J., eds. (1990), *Homosexuality/Heterosexuality: Concepts of Sexual Orientation.* New York: Oxford University Press.

Merlino, J. (1997), Support groups for professional caregivers: A role for the contemporary psychoanalyst. *J. Amer. Acad. Psychoanal.*, 25:111–122.

Miller, B. (1979), Gay fathers and their children. *Fam. Coord.*, 28:544–552.

Mississippi Gay Alliance v. Goudelock 536F.2d (1986).

Mitchell, S. (1978), Psychodynamics, homosexuality, and the question of pathology. *Psychiat.*, 41:254–263.

Mitchell, S. (1981), The psychoanalytic treatment of homosexuality: Some technical considerations. *Internat. Rev. Psycho-Anal.*, 8:63–80.

Mitchell, S. (1996), Gender and sexual orientation in the age of postmodernism: The plight of the perplexed clinician. *Gender & Psychoanal.*, 1:45–73.
Moberly, E. (1983), *Homosexuality: A New Christian Ethic.* Cambridge, UK: James Clarke.
Money, J. (1988), *Gay, Straight, and In-Between: The Sexology of Erotic Orientation.* New York: Oxford University Press.
Money, J. & Ehrhardt, A. (1972), *Man and Woman, Boy and Girl.* Baltimore, MD: Johns Hopkins University Press.
Morgenthaler, F. (1984), *Homosexuality Heterosexuality Perversion,* trans. A. Aebi. Hillsdale, NJ: The Analytic Press, 1988.
Moses, A. E, & Hawkins, R. (1982), *Counseling Lesbian Women and Gay Men: A Life Issues Approach.* St. Louis, MO: Mosby.
Moss, D. (1992), Introductory thoughts: Hating in the first person plural: The example of homophobia. *Amer. Imago,* 49:277–291.
Moss, D. (1997), On situating homophobia. *J. Amer. Psychoanal. Assn.,* 45:201–215.
Moyer, K. E. (1974), Sex differences in aggression. In *Sex Differences in Behavior,* ed. R. C. Friedman, R. M. Richart & R. L. Vande-Wiele. New York: Wiley, pp. 335–373.
National Gay & Lesbian Task Force (1997), *Legal Notes,* April 1.
Nyberg, K. L. & Alston, J. P. (1977), Analysis of public attitudes toward homosexuality. *J. Homosexual.,* 2:99–107.
O'Connor v. Donaldson, 422 US 563, 575 (1975).
O'Connor, N. & Ryan, J. (1993), *Wild Desires and Mistaken Identities: Lesbianism and Psychoanalysis.* New York: Columbia University Press.
O'Donnell, L. N., O'Donnell, C. R., Pleck, J. H. & Snarey, J. (1987), Psychosocial responses of hospital workers to acquired immune deficiency syndrome (AIDS). *J. Appl. Soc. Psychol.,* 17:269–285.
Ovesey, L. (1969), *Homosexuality and Pseudohomosexuality.* New York: Science House.
Palmore v. Sidoti, 466 US 429, 433 (1984).
Patterson, C. J. (1992), Children of lesbian and gay parents. *Child. Devel.,* 63:1025–1042.
Patterson, C. J. (1995), Lesbian mothers, gay fathers and their children. In *Lesbian, Gay and Bisexual Identities Over the Lifespan,* ed. A. R. D'Augelli & C. J. Patterson. Oxford, UK: Oxford University Press, pp. 262–293.
Patterson, C. & Chan, R. (1996), Gay fathers and their children. In *Textbook of Homosexuality and Mental Health,* ed. R. Cabaj

& T. Stein. Washington, DC: American Psychiatric Press, pp. 371–393.

Planansky, K. & Johnston, R. (1962), The incidence and relationship of homosexual and paranoid features in schizophrenia. *Brit. J. Psychiat.*, 456:604–615.

Prenzlauer, S., Drescher, J. & Winchel, R. (1992), Suicide among homosexual youth. *Amer. J. Psychiat.*, 149:1416.

Pronk, P. (1993), *Against Nature: Types of Moral Argumentation Regarding Homosexuality.* Grand Rapids, MI: Eerdmans.

Racker, H. (1968), *Transference and Countertransference.* Madison, CT: International Universities Press.

Rado, S. (1940), A critical examination of the concept of bisexuality. In *Sexual Inversion: The Multiple Roots of Homosexuality*, ed. J. Marmor. New York: Basic Books, 1965, pp. 175–189.

Rado, S. (1949), An adaptational view of sexual behavior. In *Psychosexual Development in Health and Disease*, ed. P. Hoch & J. Zubin. New York: Grune & Stratton.

Rich, C. L., Fowler, R. C., Young, D. & Blenkush, M. (1986), San Diego suicide study: Comparison of gay to straight males. *Suicide Life Threat. Behav.*, 16:448–457.

Rieker, P. & Carmen, E., eds. (1984), *The Gender Gap in Psychotherapy: Social Realities and Psychological Processes.* New York: Plenum.

Rivera, R. (1991), Sexual orientation and the law. In *Homosexuality: Research Implications for Public Policy*, ed. J. C. Gonsiorek & J. D. Weinrich. Newbury Park, CA: Sage.

Robins, E. (1981), *The Final Months: A Study of the Lives of 134 Persons Who Committed Suicide.* New York: Oxford University Press.

Romer v. Evans, 116 S. Ct. 1620 (1996).

Rosenthal, M. (1985), *The Character Factory: Baden-Powell and the Origins of the Boy Scout Movement.* New York: Pantheon.

Ross, M. W., ed. (1988), *The Treatment of Homosexuals with Mental Health Disorders.* New York: Harrington Park Press.

Roughton, R. (1995), Overcoming antihomosexual bias: A progress report. *Amer. Psychoanal.*, 29(4):15–16.

Royse, D. & Birge, B. (1987), Homophobia and attitudes towards AIDS patients among medical, nursing, and paramedical students. *Psychol. Rep.*, 61:867–870.

Rubenstein W. (1991), Challenging the military's anti-lesbian and anti-gay policy. *Law & Sexual.*, 1:239–265.

Rudolph, J. (1989), Effects of an affirmative gay psychotherapy workshop on counselors' authoritarianism. *Psychol. Rep.*, 65:945–946.

Rudolph, J. (1990), Counselors' attitudes toward homosexuality: Some tentative findings. *Psychol. Rep.*, 66:1352–1354.

Ruitenbeek, H. M. (1963), *The Problem of Homosexuality in Modern Society*. New York: Dutton.

St. Lawrence, J. S., Kelly, J. A., Owen, A. D. & Hogan, I. G. (1990), Psychologists' attitudes towards AIDS. *Psychology & Health* 4:357–365.

San Miguel, C. L. & Millham, J. (1976), The role of cognitive and situational variables in aggression toward homosexuals. *J. Homosex.*, 2:11–27.

Schafer, R. (1976), *A New Language for Psychoanalysis*. New Haven, CT: Yale University Press.

Schafer, R. (1995), The evolution of my views on nonnormative sexual practice. In: *Disorienting Sexualities*, ed. T. Domenici & R. Lesser. New York: Routledge, pp. 187–202.

Schaffner, B. (1986), Reactions of medical personnel and intimates to persons with AIDS. In *Psychotherapy and the Memorable Patient*, ed. M. Stern. New York: Haworth Press, pp. 67–80.

Schaffner B. (1990), Psychotherapy with HIV-infected persons. *New Directions for Mental Health Services*, 48:5–20.

Schaffner B. (1993), The Crucial and the Difficult Role of the Psychotherapist in the Treatment of the HIV-Positive Patient. Presented at American Academy of Psychoanalysis Meeting, San Francisco, May.

Schaffner, B. (1996), Modifying psychoanalytic methods when treating HIV-positive patients. *J. Amer. Acad. Psychoanal.*, 25:123–141.

Schwartz, D. (1993), Heterophilia—The love that dare not speak its aim. *Psychoanal. Dial.*, 3:643–652.

Sedgwick, E. (1990), *Epistemology of the Closet*. Berkeley: University of California Press.

Seeman, M. V. (1989), Resistance to specialized services for AIDS patients within psychiatry. *Hillside J. Clin. Psychiat.*, 11:17–24.

Shaffer, D. (1993), Political science. *The New Yorker*, May 3, p. 116.

Shapiro, M. F., Hayward, R. A., Guillemot, D. & Jayle, D. (1992), Residents' experiences in and attitudes toward the care of persons with AIDS in Canada, France, and the United States. *J. Amer. Med. Assn.*, 268:510–515.

Shenon, P. (1999), Pentagon moving to end abuses of "Don't ask, don't tell" policy. *The New York Times*, August 13, pp. 1, 12.
Shilts, R. (1987a), *And The Band Played On*. New York: St. Martin's Press.
Shilts, R. (1987b), In Houston, "AIDS is spelled G-A-Y." *San Francisco Chronicle*, July 30, pp. 1, 4.
Simon, M. S., Weyant, R. J., Asabigi, K. N., Zucker, L. & Koopman, J. S. (1991), Medical student attitudes toward the treatment of HIV-infected patients. *AIDS Ed. & Prev.*, 3:124–132.
Smith, M. U., Goudeau, R. E., Katner, H. P. & Farmer, J. T. (1993), Human immunodeficiency virus infection: Knowledge of the disease and attitudes towards related issues and policies among health care workers in a low-incidence nonurban hospital. *Southern Med. J.*, 86:537–544.
Socarides, C. (1968), *The Overt Homosexual*. New York: Grune & Stratton.
Socarides, C. (1978), *Homosexuality*. New York: Aronson.
Sontag, S. (1988), AIDS and its metaphors. *New York Rev. Books*, 35:(16)89–99.
Spence, D. (1982), *Narrative Truth and Historical Truth: Meaning and Interpretation in Psychoanalysis*. New York: Norton.
Stanton, M. (1991), *Sandor Ferenczi: Reconsidering Active Intervention*. Northvale, NJ: Aronson.
Stein, T. (1994), A curriculum for learning in psychiatric residencies about homosexuality, gay men, and lesbians. *Acad. Psychiat.*, 18:59–70.
Stein, T. & Cohen, C. (1986), *Contemporary Perspectives on Psychotherapy with Lesbians and Gay Men*. New York: Plenum.
Stoller, R. J. (1968), *Sex and Gender*. New York: Science House.
Stoller, R. J. (1974), Symbiosis anxiety and the development of masculinity. *Arch. Gen. Psychiat.*, 30:164–172.
Stoller, R. J. (1985), Gender identity disorders in children and adults. In *Comprehensive Textbook of Psychiatry*, Vol. 1, ed. H. I. Kaplan & B. J. Sadock. Baltimore, MD: Williams & Wilkins, pp. 1034–1041.
Sullivan, A., ed. (1997): *Same-Sex Marriage: Pro and Con*. New York: Vintage Books.
Sullivan, H. S. (1953), *The Interpersonal Theory of Psychiatry*. New York: Norton.
Sullivan, H. S. (1956), *Clinical Studies in Psychiatry*. New York: Norton.

Sulloway, F. J. (1979), *Freud: Biologist of the Mind*. New York: Basic Books.
Thompson, N., McCandless, B. P. & Strickland, B. (1971), Personal adjustment of male and female homosexuals and heterosexuals. *J. Abnorm. Psychol.*, 78:237–240.
Thornton, B (1995), The new international jurisprudence on the right to privacy: A head on collision with Bowers v. Hardwick, *Albany Law Rev.*, 58:725-725.
Townsend, M. H., Wallick, M. M. & Cambre, K. M. (1993), Gay and lesbian issues in residency training at US psychiatry programs. *Academ. Psychiat.*, 17:67–72.
United States General Accounting Office (1992), *Defense Force Management: DOD's Policy on Homosexuality*. GAO/NSAID-92-98; June.
Wallack J. J. (1989), AIDS anxiety among health care professionals. *Hosp. & Community Psychiat.* 40:507–510.
Wallick, M. M., Cambre, K. M. & Townsend, M. H. (1992), How the topic of homosexuality is taught at US medical schools. *Acad. Med.*, 67:601–603.
Walter, R. D. (1956), What became of the degenerate? A brief history of the concept. *J. Hist. Med.*, 11:422–449.
Waxler, N. (1981). Learning to be a leper: A case study in the social construction of illness. In *Social Contexts of Health, Illness and Patient Care*, ed. E. G. Mischler. New York: Cambridge University Press.
Weeks, J. (1985), *Sexuality and Its Discontents*. London: Routledge & Kegan Paul.
Weinberg, G. (1972), *Society and the Healthy Homosexual*. New York: Anchor Books.
Weinberger, M., Conover, C. J., Samsa, G. P. & Greenberg, S. M. (1992), Physicians' attitudes and practices regarding treatment of HIV-infected patients. *Southern Med. J.*, 85:683–686.
Wiedeman, G. H. (1962), Survey of psychoanalytic literature on overt male homosexuality. *J. Amer. Psychoanal. Assn.*, 10:386-409.
Wiedeman, G. H. (1974), Homosexuality: A survey. *J. Amer. Psychoanal. Assn.*, 22:651-696.
Williams, J. B. W., Rabkin, J. G., Remien, R. H., Gorman, J. M. & Ehrhardt, A. A. (1991), Multidisciplinary baseline assessment of homosexual men with and without human immunodeficiency virus infection. II. Standardized clinical assessment of current and lifetime psychopathology. *Arch. Gen. Psychiat.*, 48:124–130.

REFERENCES

Wisconsin v. Yoder, 406 US 205, 223–224 (1972).

Zucker, K. J. & Bradley, S. (1995), *Gender Identity Disorder and Psychosexual Problems in Children and Adolescents.* New York: Guilford Press.

Zucker, K. J. & Green, R. (1993), Psychological and familial aspects of gender identity disorder. *Child Adolesc. Psychiatr. Clin. North Amer.*, 2:513–543.

Index

A
Abelove, H, xiv, 78, 107
Abstinence, sexual, 33, 42
Achtenberg, R., 82, 85, 107
Acton, W., 2, 107
Adolescents, x, 18: psychotherapy with, 38–47; suicide attempts, 47–52
Adoption, 86–88
AIDS, viii, xiv, xvi, 4, 10, 50, 61, 63, 68, 105: antihomosexual bias and bias against persons with, 91–103; equated with homosexuality, 4; fear of contagion as source of, 97–98; implications for clinician, 101; nationality of health care workers and fear of, 98–99; sources of stigmatization, 102–103
AIDS patients, attitudes of house officers and nurses toward, 95; societal bias against, 91–93
Alston, J. P., 4, 118
American Academy of Pediatrics Committee on Adolescence, 42, 107
American Academy of Psychoanalysis, 106
American Association of Directors of Psychiatric Residency Training (AADPRT), view on homosexuality, 66

American Orthopsychiatric Association, 106
American Psychiatric Association (APA), vii, x, 6, 7, 8, 78, 85, 106, 107
Committee on Gay, Lesbian and Bisexual Issues, 67: removal of homosexuality from category of pathology, 7, 8
American Psychoanalytic Association, 74, 106, 107: Committee on Issues of Homosexuality, 74
American Psychological Association, 8, 80, 106: Committee on Gay and Lesbian Concerns, 27
American Public Health Association, 80
Anal penetration, fear of, 34
Antihomosexual bias (AHB): associated features, 5–6; behavior therapists and, 25; bible, condemnation in, 1; in clinical setting, 25–54; in colleges, 4; definitions and issues, 10–14; demographics related to, 5–6; discrimination, 4, 49, 62, 68, 74, 89, 100, 106; and nationality of health care workers, 98–99; historical influences in, 1–3; impact of, xvi; impact on growth and

INDEX

Antihomosexual bias *(continued)*
psychological development, 19–23; in institutions, 57–59, 82–85; laws against, 82; paranoid, psychological mechanisms in, 14–23; in psychoanalytic training, 73–76; in screening interview, 68; in society at large, 91–93; state laws outlawing, 82; in training settings, 60–73; See also Homophobia

Anxiety, ix, 18

Attitudes toward homosexuality, 3–10: of authority figures, 41–43; in boys, 19–22; of childhood peers, Little Leaguers, 20–21; of counselors, 25; in dynamic psychiatry, 6–9; in fundamentalist religion, 9–10; in general population, 3–6; among males; women's, 22

B

Baehr v. Lewin, 86, 108
Baehr v. Miike, 86, 108
Barale, M. A., xi, 107
Baumeyer, F., 108
Baumgartner, E., 101, 108
Bayer, R., 6, 7, 8, 13, 23, 78, 108
Beach, F., 23, 112
Bell, A., 33, 46, 108
Bergler, E., 7, 13, 108
Berrill, K., xiv, 5, 6, 10, 115
Berzon, B., 46, 108
Bezio v. Patenaude, 87, 108
Bias: based on sexual orientation, state laws outlawing, 82; See also Antihomosexual bias
Bieber, I., 7, 33, 73, 108
Birge, B., 93, 95, 101, 119
Bisexuality, 41–43, 45, 47, 53, 72: definitions and issues, 10–14
Blechner, M., 8, 108
Blendon, R. J., 92, 93, 108
Blumenfield, M., 98, 100, 108
Blumstein, P., 46, 108

Bonauto, M., 87, 108
Boswell, J., xi, 23, 109
Bottoms v. Bottoms, 88, 109
Bowers v. Hardwick, 79–81, 109
Boys: feminine behavior in, 39–40; attitudes toward homosexuality, 17–22
Bozett, F. W., 87, 109, 113
Bradley, S., 40, 123
Brandt, A. M., 102, 109
Bresolin, L. B., 99, 109
Brown, L. S., 28, 109
Bullough, V., 2, 78, 109
Butler, J., 26, 109
Buxton, A., 45, 109

C

Cabaj, R., xii, xiv, 9, 17, 18, 27, 33, 46, 61, 109
Cabalquinto v. Cabalquinto, 87, 109
Cambre, K. M., 62, 66, 122
Cameron, N., 16, 109
Campbell, S., 94, 96, 115
Carl, D., 46, 109
Carmen, E., xiv, 119
Center for Disease Control, 93
Chan, R., 32, 118
Chiamowitz, G. A., 95, 99, 100, 109
Child custody, 31–32, 45, 86–88
Child visitation, 45, 86–88: types of, 27–29
Clinton administration, policy on coming out in military, 84
Closet(ed), 57, 61, 62, 63, 70: faculty, closeted, 67; psychiatrists, xiv; See also "Coming out"
Coates, S., 40, 110
Cohen, C., 7, 27, 121
Colasanto, D., 4, 110
"Coming out," 18, 33, 38, 58, 70: after marriage and children, 29–31, 44–46; conflicts about, 17–18, 32–34, 41–43, 47–52; as countertransference, 37–38; educators' fear of, 67; generational differences in, 63–64, 67; on

inpatient unit, 47–50; as trainee in institutional setting, 57–59; in the workplace, 82–85; See also Closet(ed)
Confidentiality, 29, 49, 58, 59, 83
Congregation for the Doctrine of the Faith, 9–10
Conrad, F., 8, 112
Corlevale, E., 5, 110
Cort, J., 5, 110
Countertransference, 46–47, 56, 72–73, 106: in coming out, 37–38; negative, 7
Crawford. I,, 95, 99, 101, 110
Criminals, gay men and lesbians classified as, 79–82, See Sodomy laws

D
D'Augelli, A. R., 33, 94, 96, 110
Davis, C. A., 15, 116
Davison, G. C., 25, 26, 110
De Cecco, J., xiv, 23, 46, 110
Defense of Marriage Act, 86, 110
Degeneracy theory, 2
Diagnostic and Statistical Manual (DSM), x, 6, 30, 68, 73, 78: removal of homosexuality from, 69
Disability benefits, 85
Domenici, T., xiv, 8, 26, 110
Donelan, K., 92, 93, 108
Douglas, C. J., 94, 99, 100, 110
Douglas, M., 94, 102, 110
Dow, M. G., 99, 110
Downey, J., 7, 9, 17, 27, 45, 110, 112, 113
Drescher, J., xii, xv, 7, 8, 9, 26, 27, 36, 61, 73, 111, 119
DSM, See Diagnostic and Statistical Manual
Duberman, M., 2, 111
Dunlap, D., 10, 111
Dynamic psychiatry, attitudes toward homosexuality in, 6–9

E
Ego identity, 11–12, 13
Ehrhardt, A. A., 9, 12, 118, 122
Ellis, H., 13, 111
Empathic failure, 27–28, 35–38, 47–52, 94–95
Employment, antihomosexual bias in, 82–85
England v. State of Texas, 81, 111
Epstein, R. M, 98, 111
Erikson, E. H., 11, 111
Erotic attraction, defined, 11
Ethics: American Psychiatric Association guidelines related to psychiatrists in military, 85; lapses from, 28–29

F
Faculty, openly gay or lesbian, 64–65
Fag, OED definition, 21
Falco, K., 27, 111
Falk, P., 87, 112
Family psychotherapy, 38–47
Federal government, same-sex marriage and, 86; See also DOMA
Fenichel, O., 16, 17, 112
Ferenczi, S., 78, 121
Fine, G. A., 20, 112
Fisher, S. S., 7, 112
Ford, C., 23, 112
Fort, J., 8, 112
Foucault, M., 2, 26, 112
Freud, S., 13, 14, 26, 73, 78, 112
Friedman, R. C., xii, 7, 8, 9, 11, 13, 15, 17, 26, 27, 34, 40, 45, 74, 82, 110, 112, 113, 117
Frommer, M. S., 7, 113
Fundamentalist religion, attitudes in, 9–10

G
GAP, See Group for the Advancement of Psychiatry

Gay: defined, 11; identity as, 11; immigration laws, related to, 85–86; limitations on civil rights, 14
Gay, P., 7, 113
Gay patients: issues unique to treatment of, 49; psychotherapy with, 26–27, Also see AHB in clinical setting
Gebhard, P., 23, 116
Gender identity, 12, 13, 15, 22: core, 12; differentiation, 12; distinguished from sexual orientation, 13; female vs male, 19–20
Gender identity disorder (GID), of childhood, 39–40
Gender insecurity, 15
Gender role, 12, 13, 19, 37, 40, 46, 53
Georgia, sodomy laws, 79–19
Gilligan, C., 19, 113
Glunt, E. K., xiv, 92, 93, 102, 115
Goffman, E., 17, 102, 113
Golombok, S., 87, 113
Gomes, P. J., 23, 113
Gonsiorek, J. C., 2, 9, 113
Gottman, J. S., 87, 113
Green, G. D., 87, 113
Green, R., 40, 87, 113, 123
Greenberg, D., 2, 3, 7, 77, 114
Greenberg, R. P., 7, 112
Greenson, R. R., 19, 20, 114
Group for the Advancement of Psychiatry (GAP), vii, viii, ix, x, xii, xiii, 114: Committee on Adolescence, x; Committee on the College Student, xii, xiii; Committee on Cooperation with Government Agencies, x–xi; Committee on Forensic Psychiatry, ix–x; Committee on Human Sexuality, xiv–xvi, 105; Committee on Medical Education, x; Committee on Psychiatry and the Law, x; Committee on Social Issues, viii–ix; historical positions and social issues, vii–xiv; past reports relating to homosexuality, vii–xvi; publications, viii–xiii
Guitierrez, L., 79, 117

H
Halperin, D., xiv, 107
Hammersmith, S., 33, 108
Hancock, K. A., 27, 114
Hanley-Hackenbruck, P., 32, 114
Harris, A., 26, 114
Harvard Law Review, 82, 115
Harvey, J., 23, 115
Hatterer, L., 73, 115
Hawaii, supreme Court, ruling on same-sex marriage, 86
Hawkins, R., 88, 118
Health care professionals, antihomosexual bias and AIDS bias in, 93–97, 103: cultural aspects of, 98–99
Health insurance benefits, 85
Helminiak, D., 23, 115
Hendin, H., 9, 115
Henry, K., 94, 96, 115
Herek, G. M., xiv, 3, 5, 6, 10, 13, 92, 93, 102, 115
"Heterocentrism," 3
Heterosexism, 2, 3, 13, 18, 28, 30–31, 35, 49, 69–70, 74–75
Heterosexual orientation, 11
Heterosexuality: as treatment goal, 48; definitions and issues, 10–14;
HIV, xvi, 34, 62, 91–103, See also AIDS
Hirschfeld, M., 78
Holt, R. R., 7, 115
Homophobia, 14, 16, 31, 96: defined, 13; external, 13; internalized, 13, 17–18, 28, 36, 44, 49–50; origins of, 13; See also Antihomosexual bias
Homosexual orientation, 11
Homosexual/heterosexual binary, 2

INDEX

Homosexuality: attitudes toward, 3–10; as character pathology, 74; etiology of, 7; GAP reports relating to, vii–xvi; identified as treatable illness, xi, 6; issues, 10–14; negative perceptions of, 1–3; normal variant model of, 2–3; prediction of, 39–40; as security risk, xi; sin to illness, 1–2
Hooker, E., 7, 23, 69, 115
Horowitz, W. A., 15, 116
Hunter, C. E., 96, 115
Hunter, N., 87, 115

I
Indiana University, Institute for Sex Research, 3
Isay, R., xv, 7, 8, 11, 27, 73, 74, 116

J
Johnson, R., 15, 119
Jones, E. 73
Jones, F., 13, 84, 116

K
Kalman, C. M., 94, 99, 100, 110
Kalman, T. P., 94, 99, 100, 110
Kiersky, S., 26, 116
Kinsey, A., xi, 10, 23, 116
Kirkpatrick, M., 32, 76, 87, 88, 116
Klaf, F. S., 15, 116
Klassen, A. P., 3, 116
Klein, H. R., 15, 116
Kleinman, A., 91, 116
Klinger, R. L., 5, 116
Knox, M. D., 99, 110
Koshes, R., 13, 84, 116
Krafft-Ebing, R., 2, 13, 116
Kwawer, J., 7, 117

L
Laws/legislation: Appeal in Pima City Juvenile Action, 81, 108; Colorado, "Amendment Two", 81; Helms amendment, 93; legislation for gay rights, 93; state laws outlawing discrimination based on sexual orientation, 82

Legal aspects of antihomosexual bias and mental health, 77–89: custody, adoption, procreation, and visitation, 86–88; institutions and employment, 82–85; marriage and spousal benefits, 85–86; privacy and rights of association, 79–82

Lesbian: couple, 47; defined, 11; gender identification and sexual orientation in, 22; identity as, 11, 22, 36–37; immigration laws and, 85–86; mother, 75–76, 86–88; patients, antihomosexual attitudes of, 18
Lesser, R., xiv, 8, 26, 110, 117
Levenson, E., 25, 26, 56, 117
Levitt, E. E., 3, 116
Lewes, K., 6, 7, 8, 73, 78, 117
Lief, H., 8, 74, 117
Lilling, A., 8, 26, 74, 113, 117

M
Magee, M., xv, 7, 8, 11, 26, 27, 73, 117
Marmor, J., xiv, 7, 27, 74, 117
Marriage: coming out in context of, 44–46; same-sex, legal aspects, 85–86
Martin, C., xi, 11, 23, 116
Masturbation, as putative cause of homosexuality, 2
Mattison, A., 46, 117
McCandless B. P., 88, 122
McCrary, I., 79, 117
McWhirter, D, xii, 46, 117
Medical school: antihomosexual bias in, 58–59, 62–66; student–faculty groups, gay and lesbian, 63–64

Medical students: absence of gay and lesbian role models, 63–64; attitudes toward AIDS patients, 96–97; educating about gay and lesbian health issues, 64–66; organizing conference on homosexuality, 58–59; prejudice against gay and lesbian, 59–60
Mental disorder, removal of homosexuality as, 7–8
Merlino, J., 56, 117
Military, antihomosexual bias in, 7, 82–85
Miller, B., 97, 117
Miller, D., xv, 7, 8, 11, 26, 27, 73, 117
Millham, J., 6, 120
Minorities, health care workers, AHB and fear of AIDS in, 98
Misattribution, 27; See also stereotyping, stigma
Mississippi Gay Alliance v. Goudelock, 81, 117
Mitchell, S., 7, 117
Moberly, E., 23, 118
Money, J., 11, 12, 118
Morgenthaler, F., 74, 118
Moses, A. E., 88, 118
Moss, D., 14, 118
Moyer, K. E., 6, 118

N
National Association of Social Workers, 8, 106
National Gay & Lesbian Task Force, 86, 118
National Opinion Research Center, 3
Neutrality, therapeutic, 26, 45, 56–57; abandonment of, 7, 29–31
Nuclear family, idealization of, 2
Nyberg, K. L., 4, 118

O
Objectivity, loss of, 72; See also countertransference

O'Connor, N., 7, 8, 118
O'Connor v. Donaldson, 80, 118
O'Donnell, L. N., 94, 95, 118
Ovesey, L., 16, 73, 118

P
Palmore v. Sidoti, 80, 118
Parents: attitudes and expectations, 42, 48; gay and lesbian, 31–32; sexual orientation of, 45
Parker, D., 23, 110
Pathologizing type of antihomosexual bias, 27, 58–59, 60, 66, 69–70, 73–74
Patient, antihomosexual bias toward gay doctor, 71–72
Patient care, for AIDS patient, impact of antihomosexual bias on, 99–101
Patterson, C. J., 32, 33, 110, 118
Pensions, spousal, 85
Phobic, psychological mechanisms, antihomosexual bias, 16–17, See also Homophobia
Planansky, K., 15, 119
Pomeroy, W., xi, 10, 23, 116
Prejudice, racial and sexual, viii, ix, xiv, xvi, 4, 11, 13, 18, 56, 57, 67
Prenzlauer, S., 9, 119
President's Commission on AIDS, 93
Privacy: legal aspects of, 79–82; patient-physician, in military, 83
Procreation rights, 86–88
Pronk, P., 23, 119

Q
Quality in health care, for HIV-positive patients, 100

R
Racker, H., 25, 119
Rado, S., 33, 73, 119
Reinisch, J., xii, 117
Religion of health care workers, AHB and fear of AIDS and, 98

INDEX

Religious beliefs and values in interfacing with AIDS patients, 4, 34, 37, 48, 49, 50–52, 53
Residency training, antihomosexual bias in, 66–73
Rich, C. L., 9, 119
Rieker, P., xiv, 119
Right of association, 79–82
Rivera, R., 83, 119
Robins, E., 9, 119
Role models, 57, 70: absence in training, 46, 63–64, 70–71; adolescent identification with, 52
Romer v. Evans, 81, 119
Rosenthal, M., 2, 119
Ross, M. W., 27, 96, 115, 119
Roughton, R., 74, 119
Roy, R., 32, 87, 88, 116
Royse, D., 93, 95, 101, 119
Rubenstein, W., 82, 83, 119
Rudolph, J., 8, 25, 120
Ruitenbeek, H. M., 7, 120
Rutter, M., 87, 113
Ryan, J., 7, 8, 118

S
St. Lawrence, J. S., 95, 96, 97, 116, 120
San Miguel, C. L., 6, 120
Sanders, S., xii, 117
Scapegoating, 22
Schafer, R., 26, 56, 120
Schaffner, B., 101, 120
School Desegregation Report, viii
Schwartz, D., 26, 120
Schwartz, P., 46, 108
Sedgwick, E., 26, 120
Seeman, M. V., 94, 102, 120
Self-esteem, ix, 17, 19, 31; masculine, 20; medical students, 62
Self-hatred, antihomosexual, 28
Sexual orientation, 22, 28, 38, 45, 47, 56, 69, 82: adolescent confusion about, 41–43; defined, 11; disclosure of, 17–18; distinguished from gender identity, 13; prediction of, 40; state laws outlawing discrimination based on, 82; of supervisor, 67; unsolicited attempts at changing, 28, 35–36; See also "Coming out"
Shaffer, D., 9, 120
Shame: erotic feelings and, 42–43; HIV and, 101; internalized homophobia and, 18
Shapiro, M. F., 100, 120
Shenon, P., 84, 121
Shilts, R., 92, 93, 121
Simon, M. S., 98, 121
Smith, L., 87, 113
Smith, M. U., 95, 99, 121
Smith, S., Jr., 96, 116
Socarides, C., 7, 10, 13, 73, 121
Social security benefits, 85
Sodomy laws, 79–81
Sontag, S., 91, 92, 102, 121
Spence, D., 26, 56, 121
Spencer, A., 87, 113
Spousal benefits, legal aspects of, 85–86
Stanton, M., 78, 121
Stein, T. S., xii, xiv, 5, 7, 9, 17, 18, 27, 33, 46, 61, 67, 109, 116, 121
Steiner, C. M., 8, 112
Stereotypes/stereotyping, ix–x, xii, 6, 22, 27, 31–34, 43–44, 46–47, 52–53, 59–60, 61
Stigma, 3, 11, 14, 17, 27, 28, 34, 59, 61, 66, 93, 103
Stoller, R. J., 12, 19, 20, 74, 121
Strickland, B., 88, 122
Students, gay or lesbian, xiii, 68; See also Medical Students
Suicide/suicide attempts, 9, 18, 37–38, 47–52, 50–52
Sullivan, A., 85, 121
Sullivan, H. S., 16, 121
Sulloway, F. J., 7, 122
Supervision, 29–31: impact of antihomosexual bias on, 55–76

Supervisor: gay and lesbian, 58; identifying with, 55–56; sexual orientation of, 67; unrecognized bias in, 57

Supervisor–supervisee relationship, power differential in, 59–60

T

Tax benefits, 85

Therapist: antihomosexual countertransference in, 35–36, 46–47; gay and lesbian, 8, 36–38; lack of knowledge related to homosexuality, 38–39, 46–47; openly gay, xiii, 8; training in gay and lesbian issues, xiv

Thompson, N., 88, 122

Thornton, B., 79, 122

Tomboys, 22–23

Townsend, M. H., 62, 66, 122

Training, training programs: inservice, 52–53; impact of antihomosexual bias in, 73–76; psychoeducation of hospital staff, 52–55; AHB in, 73–76; See also Residency training

U

United States General Accounting Office, 82, 83, 84, 122

United States Senate, 93

U. S. Supreme Court, rulings on antihomosexual bias, 79–82

V

Victorianism, antisexual, 2

Violence, antigay, 4, 5, 6, 9–10, 14, 93

W

Wallack, J. J., 94, 95, 98, 99, 100, 101, 122

Wallick, M. M., 62, 66, 122

Walter, R. D., 2, 122

Waxler, N., 92, 122

Weeks, J., 2, 122

Weinberg, G., xiv, 13, 122

Weinberg, M., 33, 46, 108

Weinberger, M., 101, 122

Weinrich, J. D., 9, 113

Wiedeman, G. H., 6, 122

Williams, C. J., 3, 116

Williams, J. B. W., 9, 122

Willinbring, K., 94, 96, 115

Wilson, G. T., 25, 26, 110

Winchel, R., 9, 119

Wisconsin v. Yoder, 80, 123

Wolfe, S., 40, 110

Z

Zucker, K. J., 40, 123